GIRLS' SCOLIOSIS:
WHY MORE GIRLS ARE AFFECTED THAN
BOYS?
THE CAUSE, PREVENTION AND
TREATMENTS

TAKE CARE OF YOUR SPINE,
IT IS THE BACKBONE OF GOOD HEALTH,
BEARING AND SPLENDOR

**do not delay, start the scoliosis treatment with
the right exercises when the abnormal curve of
scoliosis is still small and easier to correct.**

BY   S.ELIA

The "do not delay campaign" of the famous orthopedic surgeon Dr. John H. Moe 1905-1988 , that was my inspiration to write about scoliosis and the spinal active flexion exercises.

"Dr.. 'John H. Moe 1905-1988 a University of Minnesota orthopedic surgeon, who founded the Scoliosis Research Society in 1966 and he began a "do not delay" campaign for scoliosis, and he wrote " procrastination was the most pernicious problem in idiopathic scoliosis and sad to see a child come with a severe curve requiring surgery with X-rays taken many years before showing a mild curve that could have been easily treated with a brace.46'Dangerous Curve" campaign "

Disclaimer:

This book is for information ONLY and is not intended to serve as medical advice. Anyone seeking specific advice or assistance should consult his or her doctor. If they do not like the advice of their doctor they should seek a second opinion from another doctor. You should always work with the advise and blessing of your trusted doctor. Any time there is pain and stiffness of the spine accompanied with chills or fever see a doctor immediately for proper medical diagnosis and treatments.

NB. The exercises described in this book are good for anyone that has a spine for the prevention and treatment of scoliosis. However these exercises are not INTENDED for people with spinal pathology, fractures , surgery with fusion and rods in their spines. If that's your situation consult your trusted doctor before you start any strenuous exercises.

THE AUTHOR

S.ELIA

DEDICATION

I dedicate this book to all those girls and others
that are affected with idiopathic scoliosis and do
not know what to do to stop the progression of
their abnormal spinal curve. It is my hope that this
book will help them find some answers to their
questions and perhaps the help they need for
their scoliosis.

 It is also dedicated to all those mothers that worry
about their kid's health when they are first
diagnosed with scoliosis. By encouraging   and
supervising their youngsters to do   the S.A.F.E.

exercises daily, will give them hope and eliminate their anguish and frustration when they see their kids getting better and have a healthy, strong and flexible spine.

TABLE OF CONTENTS

@@@@@@@@@@@@@

1)Introduction.

In this book we are going to talk about why more girls are affected with scoliosis than boys. The scoliosis cause , the diagnosis, treatments and prevention of scoliosis.
Although the title of this book is " GIRLS' SCOLIOSIS", the content in this book is about scoliosis in general, the abnormal spinal curve that affects people of all ages and all genders. I chose this title because more girls are affected by scoliosis than boys and there is a specific reason why girls have scoliosis more often than boys of the same age.
In my previous books I described the main causes and new classification of the idiopathic scoliosis and ways to prevent and treat scoliosis with the spinal exercises.
 In this book I will try to explain in detail why the girls are more vulnerable to be affected with scoliosis and ways to stop the progression of the abnormal spinal curve. I will describe how to prevent scoliosis and especially in girls and ways to check and recognize scoliosis , what exercise to do and when you should see your doctor for proper diagnosis and treatments. Scoliosis is a

preventable condition and it can be treated successfully with the proper spinal exercises at home especially in the early stages when the abnormal curve is still small!   Anybody can recognized a crooked spine , the so called scoliosis, but the proper diagnosis of scoliosis is done by taking x-rays of the spine AP   and lateral to see what type of scoliosis is and see if there is any pathology present causing the abnormal curve. The sooner the scoliosis is diagnosed the better chances are to stop the progression of the curve and even reverse it with exercises. A delay in diagnosing the abnormal curve there is danger that the scoliosis become severe that would require   surgery to correct it.

There is an old wise proverb saying, that expresses an obvious truth and often offers advice :
" A stitch in time saves nine".   In the case of scoliosis the earliest the diagnosis is made, the better the chances to stop the progression of the abnormal curve and with good chances to reverse it with exercises.

@@@@@@@@@@@@@@@@@@@@@@@@
@@@@@@

2)The main reasons why girls are affected with scoliosis.

For years the scientific community could not understand why girls are affected more often with idiopathic scoliosis than boys and what was the

cause of the idiopathic scoliosis in general.
There are many theories out there about the cause
of idiopathic scoliosis and in particular about girls
that they have a sudden spurt of skeletal growth .
There are theories , talking about genes,
hereditary, selenium , copper deficiencies etc. .One
particular theory theorize that the bones of girls
grow faster than the nerves and the nerves pull the
bones into an abnormal curve, called scoliosis.
Fortunately all those theories are just that ,
theories, and not a proven fact. If that was a proven
fact when the spinal surgeons straighten surgically
the spine and put rods to hold the spine straight, if
the nerves were short, the nerves would break and
cause a catastrophic paralysis from the broken
nerves. Something which fortunately never
happens and the spinal nerves work perfectly with
most spinal surgeries and have good results.
The reason that the girls are affected with scoliosis
more often than the boys is due to their motherly
instinct. The girls want to prepare themselves for
the moment that all girls secretly desire, when they
will have kids of their own, when they become
mothers themselves. From the moment that are able
to walk they like to play with dolls fantasizing that
the dolls are their kids. When they are older they
like to play with younger kids, their siblings,
nieces and nephews or the neighbors kids or any
kids that are available. In their effort to prepare

and hone their skills for motherhood by lifting and carrying younger kids around they suffer injuries to their spine and pelvic joints. These injuries usually go unnoticed and untreated and cause an abnormal side curve in the low back and an apparent short leg. With time the body tries to straighten up and bring the centre of gravity inside the base of the body which is the feet. In order to bring the centre of gravity inside the base of the body, a second curve is formed higher up in the spine thus forming an S type scoliosis which is the most common type of scoliosis affected by girls. The other type of idiopathic scoliosis is the C type which most of the time is caused by bad postural positions, when they lean to one side all the time when they sit, work or carry heavy objects on one side of their body. If the C type of scoliosis is not corrected it will eventually become an S type of scoliosis in an attempt of the body to bring the centre of gravity inside the base of the body, the two feet, when they are in the standing position. That is the righting reflex of the human body.

In short the reason why girls are affected with scoliosis more often than the boys, is their motherhood instinct and their effort to prepare for their future role of being mothers. The lifting and carrying around heavy kids causes lifting injuries in the lumbar-sacral area and the beginning of scoliosis.

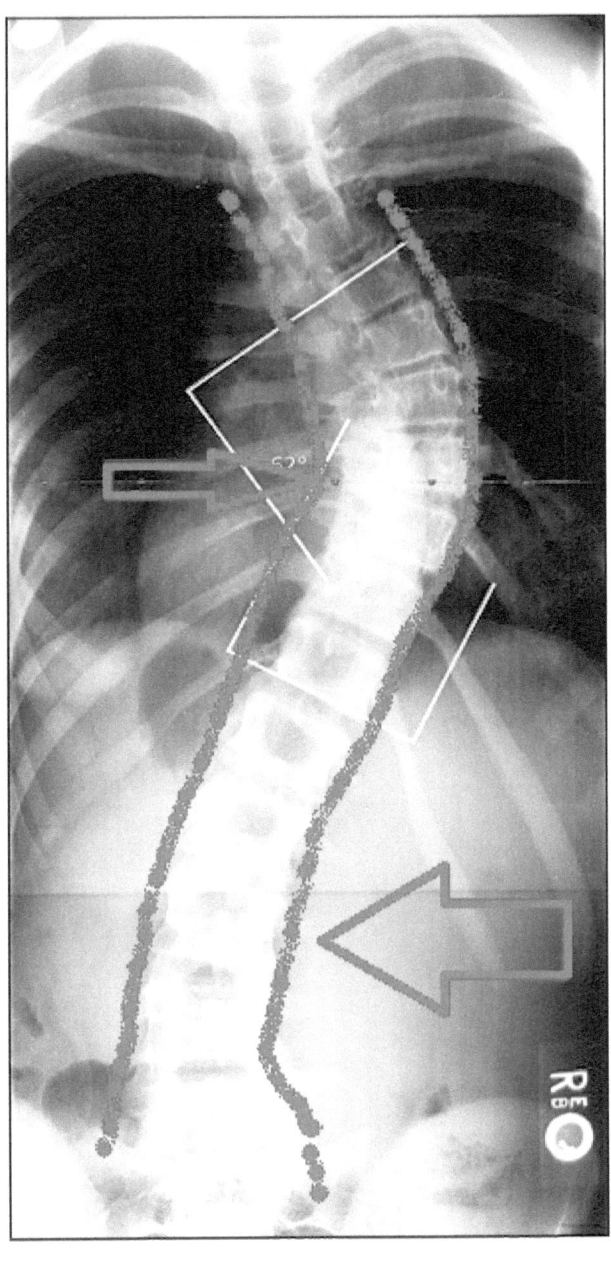

@@@@@@@@@@@@@@@@@@@@@@@@
@@@@@@@

3)What is scoliosis.

Scoliosis is an abnormal curve of the human spine to the side, either to the left or right side.
There are many types of scoliosis and are named after their cause.

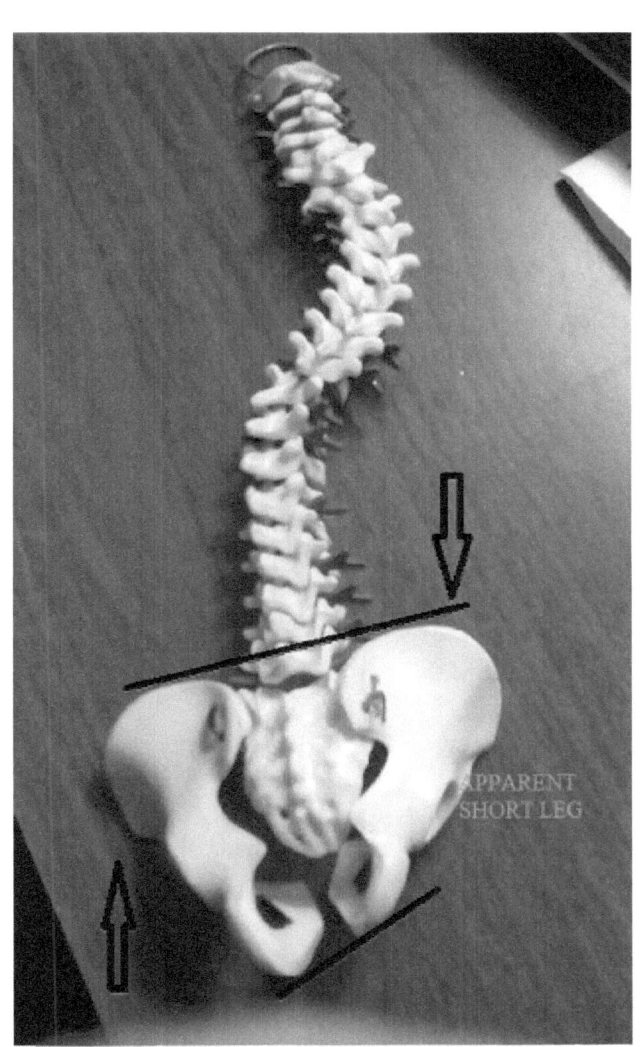

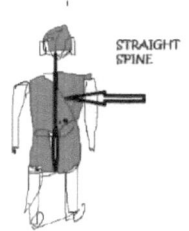
STRAIGHT
SPINE

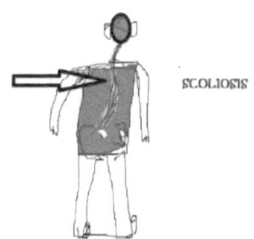
SCOLIOSIS

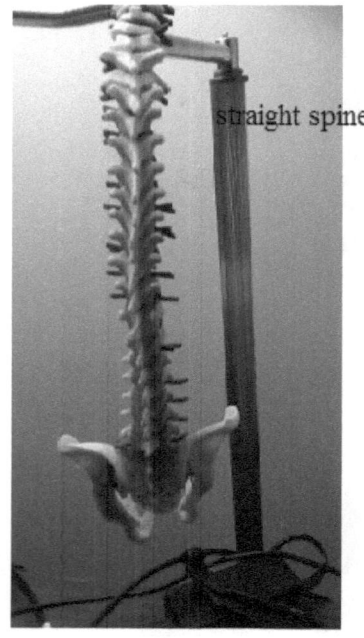
straight spine

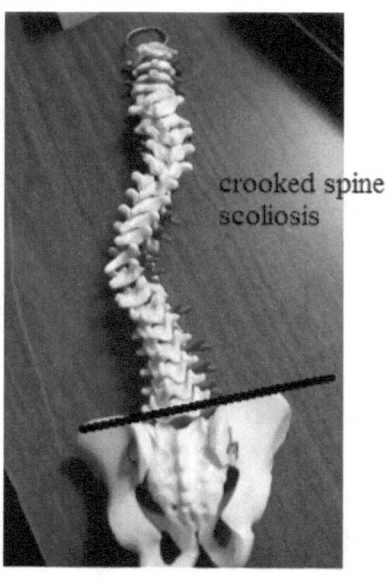
crooked spine
scoliosis

@@@@@@@@@@@@@@@@@@@@@@@@@
@@@@@@@

4)TYPES OF SCOLIOSIS.

There are two types of scoliosis:
 a) congenital
 and b) acquired.

a) the congenital scoliosis :

The congenital scoliosis is present before the baby
is born and it is developed while the baby was in
the mother's womb.
The congenital scoliosis is the worst type of
scoliosis and it is very difficult to treat. The bones
of the spine are usually malformed, fused together,
or half developed forming acute angles causing
severe abnormal curves . This type of scoliosis is
treated by the specialist orthopedic and
neurosurgeons .

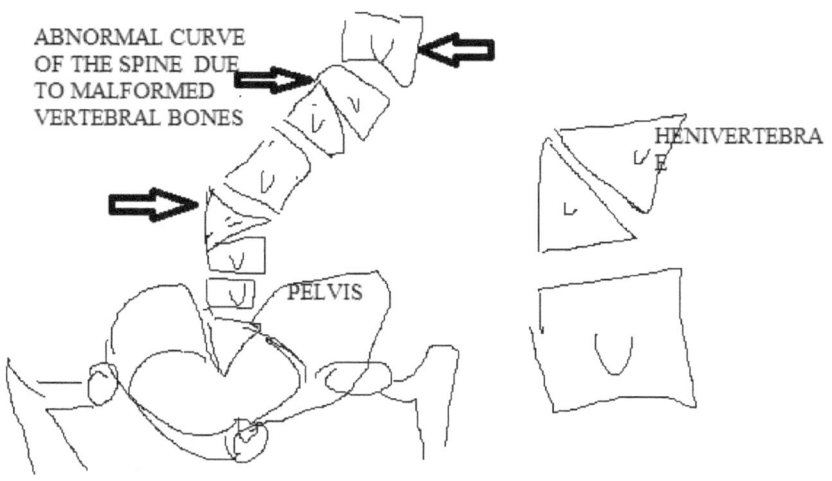

CONGENITAL SCOLIOSIS DUE TO MALFORMED BONES

THIS TYPE OF SCOLIOSIS IS VERY DIFFICULT TO TREAT

ABNORMAL CURVE OF THE SPINE DUE TO MALFORMED VERTEBRAL BONES

HEMIVERTEBRA

PELVIS

For years the scientific community did not know the cause of the congenital scoliosis and they were doing the best they could to treat this abnormal spinal curve with observation, surgery, braces and exercises with limited success due to the severity of the abnormal curve.

But a new research done by a British scientist found that The causative factor for such abnormalities to the spine and other malformations to the unborn baby, such as cleft palate and cleft lips, might be nutritional

deficiencies during pregnancy such as folic acid .
And I quote from his published research: "We
already know that **folic acid** reduces the risk of
neural tube defects, including spinal bifida. Our
research suggests that **folic acid** also helps **prevent**
facial **clefts**, another common birth defect." Jan 26,
2007Allen J. Wilcox, M.D., Ph.D., lead NIEHS
author on the new study published online in the
British Medical Journal. "

His research suggest that other abnormalities of
the spine , such as spinal bifida and spinal neural
abnormalities might be prevented when the
pregnant mothers take folic acid during their
pregnancy.

The recommended daily dietary allowance for
folate (folic acid) for adults is 400 micrograms or
0.4 mg.

Many doctors now recommend folic acid to the
pregnant women to prevent some types of
malformations.

Any woman contemplating to have babies should
talk with their doctor about folic acid
supplementation to prevent any possible
abnormalities and malformations to her babies.

There might be other nutritional deficiencies or
exposure to chemical or environmental substances
not yet identified that can cause deformities to the
unborn child including congenital scoliosis.

Finally there is also a possibility that abnormal

spermatozoa of the father might have some abnormality due to nutritional deficiencies , chemical , physical or environmental substances that might contribute to the congenital scoliosis and other baby malformations which we do not know yet.

Anyway the British research identified the folic acid as the causative factor in the congenital scoliosis and other malformations , and that's a good start.

Any woman contemplating to have babies should talk with her doctor about folic acid supplementation to prevent any possible abnormalities to her babies.

Any couple that want to have healthy kids they should take the necessary precautions to avoid any damage to their unborn child.

Both parents the father and the future mother should have good nutritional diet so they can provide all the necessary nutrients that the baby needs to be healthy. A consultation with the family doctor will provide the necessary information about good nutrition and any supplements that might be needed.

They should also avoid smoking, drinking and illicit drugs which can cause damage to the unborn child. Many times kids are born with symptoms of alcohol and drug symptoms.

*https://www.addictionhelper.com/**children/born-with-addiction-why**-and-how-it-is-treated*

***Children born** addicted to **drugs, children** suffering from withdrawal, **alcohol and drugs**. When a baby has been exposed to **drugs** in the womb there is a risk that the baby may become passively addicted to the **drugs** the mother is taking."*

Even prescription drugs can cause damage and abnormalities to the unborn children, like the

*https://www.englishonline.at/health_medicine/**thalidomide/thalidomide**-victims.htm*

"Thalidomide is a drug that caused one of the greatest medical scandals in history, in which

thousands of babies around the world were malformed.."

A planned pregnancy with all the necessary precautions , good nutrition and any necessary supplements can have a good chance to produce healthy children and happy parents.

If the congenital scoliosis is not diagnosed at birth or early childhood ,it will lead to severe spinal scoliosis later on in life which will require surgery or multiple surgeries and or braces.

The congenital scoliosis is best diagnosed and treated by the orthopedic child specialists.

b) Acquired scoliosis:

When the abnormal spinal curve develops after birth, then it is called acquired scoliosis,   has many causes and is classified according to the causative factor and the age of the patient:

1) Traumatic scoliosis, due to an injury to the spine causing the abnormal curve . Can occur at any time. it is an emergency and is treated in a hospital by the specialist.
2) pathological scoliosis due to some pathology on

the spine, like tumors, fracture, infections, etc . can occur at any time and is treated in a hospital by specialists.

3)Degenerative scoliosis results from degenerative changes or collapsed vertebrae of the spine which usually is found in older people.

4) neuromuscular scoliosis from abnormalities of the central nervous system or muscles disease, like cerebral palsy, muscular atrophy etc

The above four acquired types of scoliosis are best treated by the orthopedic specialist and neurologists and we will not discuss them any further in this book.

5) The Idiopathic scoliosis which apparently has no known cause and occurs during the growing years of the youngsters. This is the type of scoliosis we will discuss in this book.

The idiopathic scoliosis is classified according to the age of the patient.

A) infantile idiopathic scoliosis 0 to 3 years old

B) juvenile idiopathic scoliosis ages 4 to 9

C) adolescent idiopathic scoliosis ages 9 to 20

D) adult idiopathic scoliosis when the abnormal curve develops after age 20.

If the child was normal and free of any abnormal spinal curves at birth then there must be a real cause for that abnormal curve called idiopathic scoliosis , to develop. And that's what we are going to explore in this book, causes, diagnosis, prevention and treatments .

For too long the scientific community has been stuck with that archaic name, idiopathic scoliosis, since the era of Hippocrates , meaning that they do not know the cause of the abnormal curve. The patients are not served well with that definition of idiopathic scoliosis which develops mostly during the growing years of the youngsters . When the doctors diagnose this type of scoliosis, they throw their hands up in the air saying , "we can not do anything about it, we do not know the cause" and "we will wait and see what happens in the future" and that's not good enough for the youngsters which their spinal curve will get worse as the time goes by and with that advice. Eventually they send them to an orthopedic specialist for evaluation but by then the abnormal curve is getting worse.

THERE IS AN URGENT NEED TO RE-CLASSIFY THE IDIOPATHIC SCOLIOSIS, TO IDENTIFY THE REAL CAUSE OF THE SCOLIOSIS, REMOVE THE CAUSE FOR BETTER RESULTS

WITH   ANY TREATMENT INCLUDING THE SPINAL EXERCISES.

5)THE IDIOPATHIC SCOLIOSIS   RE-CLASSIFICATION

After   taking a closer look of the so called idiopathic scoliosis and exploring all plausible causes of the abnormal curve I re-classify the idiopathic scoliosis as follows.

1)idiopathic scoliosis 0-3 years old   to re-classify to the plausible causes:

a) <u>positional infantile scoliosis</u>. The abnormal curve is caused by the position they hold the baby and the way the baby sleeps. Sleeping face down will have an upper thoracic and cervical abnormal curve(scoliosis) and or skull and face malformation, called <u>positional plagiocephaly</u>, due the fact that the baby's skull is very soft at that age and can easily be malformed.

b)<u>traumatic infantile scoliosis</u>: from some kind of injury to the young spine. From   accidental falls, tantrum fits, abnormal hugging when the child tries to escape a hug or bear hugs, neglect , or

even tight baby clothing which the care givers
trying forcibly to dress or undress the little one
and can result in injuries to neck, pelvis and feet.
The result might be pointed in feet , or pointed out
feet, or walking with a limb. Parents should try to
give the kids comfortable clothing and properly fit
shoes and be gentle with the little ones.

 2) _juvenile idiopathic scoliosis _ages 4 to 9   re-
classified due to the plausible causes of this
abnormal spinal curve.

a)_postural juvenile scoliosis _: caused by poor
postural habits , slouching while sitting , walking ,
playing video games, watching television etc.

b) _baby-sitting juvenile scoliosis_:

This is the main reason why more girls are affected
with scoliosis.

The mother instinct that all girls have to prepare
for motherhood, playing with dolls and when they
are older playing with babies, lifting , hugging
and carrying them around. The babies are too
heavy for them causing them strain and injuries to
their spine and pelvic joints   thus the beginning of
the abnormal spinal curve , called scoliosis.
In reality this type of scoliosis is a lifting and
twisting injury to the low back and sacroiliac
joints. I call it baby-sitting which   occurs while
baby-sitting or playing with younger kids.

c)*traumatic juvenile scoliosis:*
This type of scoliosis is caused by accidental falls from falling down or while playing causing injuries to their sacrum-pelvic-lumbar area causing an apparent false short leg thus creating the perfect condition for a compensatory scoliosis above the injury.
This type of injury is usually unreported and untreated because the child did not report it.
d) *Short leg juvenile scoliosis* when there is a true short leg causing an imbalance to the pelvis and the spine creating an abnormal lumbar spinal curve to compensate for the short leg. Later on a secondary compensatory curve occurs in the thoracic spine due to the righting reflex.

3) *adolescent idiopathic scoliosis* ages 9 to 20 years old. To be re-classified the same as the previous juvenile classification as the causes are basically the same.

a)*postural adolescent scoliosis :* caused by poor postural habits , slouching while sitting , walking , playing video games, watching television etc.
b) baby-sitting adolescent scoliosis:
This is the main reason why more girls are affected with scoliosis.
The mother instinct that all girls have to prepare

for motherhood, playing with dolls and when they are older playing with real babies, lifting, hugging and carrying them around. The babies are too heavy for them causing them strain and injuries to their spine and pelvic joints thus the beginning of the abnormal spinal curve, scoliosis.

c)traumatic adolescent scoliosis:
This type of scoliosis is caused by accidental falls from falling down or while playing causing injuries to their sacrum-pelvic-lumbar area causing an apparent false short leg thus creating the perfect condition for a lumbar scoliosis and a compensatory scoliosis above the injury. This injury can happen from lifting heavy objects. This type of injury is usually unreported and untreated because the child did not report it.
d) Short leg adolescent scoliosis when there is a true short leg causing an imbalance to the pelvis and the spine creating an abnormal spinal curve.

4) adult idiopathic scoliosis, when the abnormal curve develops after age 20.
This type of idiopathic scoliosis should be re-classified according to the plausible causes of the abnormal spinal curve called scoliosis.
a) postural adult scoliosis : caused by

poor postural habits , slouching while sitting , walking , playing video games, watching television etc.

b)*traumatic adult scoliosis* :This type of scoliosis is caused by accidental falls from falling down or while bending down to lift something , even a pencil, causing injuries to their sacrum-pelvic-lumbar area causing an apparent false short leg, thus creating the perfect condition for a compensatory scoliosis above the injury. They can have injuries to the spine from playing contact sports , horsing around or even a violent BEAR HUG from a friend or a teammate something which I wrote about it in my book " THE PROS AND CONS OF THE HUMAN HUG " . by S.ELIA and Published by amazon.com. They might have repeated injuries to the low back and had an ineffective treatments.

c)*occupational adult scoliosis*.

This type of scoliosis is the result of awkward positioning while working. Fortunately with the new ergonomics this type of scoliosis is less prevalent, but still can happen when they work day in day out in an awkward position .

6)To conclude and summarize .

One might think that there are a lot of causes and names for the scoliosis, but in reality there can be condensed into only just three causes , or a combination of the following three, of the so called idiopathic scoliosis.

<u>1) postural scoliosis</u>, from poor habitual postural positions, when prolong sitting, standing or lying down as in the case of babies (positional scoliosis) when they hold them and they put them to sleep on the same position.

<u>2) traumatic scoliosis</u>, from some sort of injury, strain or sprain in the low back , sacroiliac joints, from lifting or twisting, causing an apparent short leg and the creation of primary low back scoliosis and a secondary compensatory spinal curve in the thoracic area to compensate for the low back spinal curve. This is the body's attempt to bring the centre of gravity within the base of the body, the two feet. That is the so called righting reflex.

<u>The righting reflex, is a reflex that correct the orientation of the body when it is taken out of its normal upright</u>

position.

3) _A true short leg scoliosis_, when there is
a true short leg which causes an imbalance in the
pelvic region creating an abnormal lumbar area
curve in the spine, scoliosis, and a compensatory
curve in the thoracic region. Again due to the
righting reflex.

That's it, just three major causes or a combination
of the three. Any attempt to prevent or treat
scoliosis, you have to correct the above three
causes in order to stop the progression of the
abnormal curve, called scoliosis, and even reverse
it back to normal.
In the absence of the above three causes , the spine
does not have any chance to develop any
abnormal curve, the so called scoliosis, idiopathic
or any other name.
And the successful removal of the above causes of
scoliosis, especially when in the early stages, the
abnormal curve should be eliminated and the spine
will return back to its normal straight condition.
That is why it is very important to identify and
remove or correct the above three causes , and
when that is done the spine will return back to its
normal position.
No treatment , can have   any success without

identifying and the removal of the above three causes. <u>That's the major reason why many types of conservative treatments fail to reverse scoliosis, because they fail to identify and remove what is causing that scoliosis they are trying to correct. No matter what you do , if you do not identify and remove the   cause and the cause is still there, it will continue to make the abnormal curve to return and get worse.</u>

Somebody, put it this way, FIND THE CAUSE, FIX THE CAUSE AND THE PATIENT WILL DO WELL!!!

The scientific and the health care community can take a look at the re-classification of the so called idiopathic scoliosis and they can either adopt the new names for   the idiopathic scoliosis or they can come up with their own re-classification   to serve the people with scoliosis better , especially the youngsters when they are first diagnosed with a mild scoliosis. The status quo of the " wait and see approach " or " the observation period ," "as it is called now, it is not working well for the affected youngsters . On the contrary it works against them and a mild scoliosis which can be treated   with spinal exercises to stop the progression of the abnormal curve, is left untreated and gets worse. The   archaic name idiopathic scoliosis has been around from the ancient times *and it is about time to give this condition new names according to the plausible causes and by just removing the plausible causes the patients will get better. With the right spinal exercises, will get them well, like the millions of athletes that exercise daily and they have no scoliosis!*

To "the wait and see approach "
I have to agree with Dr.. 'John H. Moe 1905-1988 a University of Minnesota orthopedic surgeon, who founded the Scoliosis Research Society in 1966 and he began a "do not delay" campaign for scoliosis, and he wrote "procrastination was the most pernicious problem in idiopathic scoliosis and sad to see a child come with a severe curve requiring surgery with X-rays taken many years before showing a mild curve that could have been easily treated with a brace.46'Dangerous Curve" campaign
The wait and see approach or as is now called "OBSERVATION PERIOD" I suggest to replace it with "THE ACTION TO STOP THE ABNORMAL CURVE OF SCOLIOSIS FROM GETTING WORSE" . By removing the cause or in other words the bad habits of the youngsters, the lifting of babies or other heavy objects that cause the scoliosis to get worse, and with the spinal active flexion exercises, in short S.A.F.E.

the patients will get better.

The archaic name, idiopathic scoliosis has been around from the ancient times and it is about time to give this condition new names according to the plausible causes and by just removing the plausible causes the patients will get better. With the spinal exercises will get them well, like the millions of athletes that exercise daily and they have no scoliosis!

Millions of people are diagnosed with mild scoliosis every year and with the existing protocol of treating scoliosis, especially the "WAIT AND SEE APPROACH" or the so called "OBSERVATION PERIOD" their scoliosis will progress to severe scoliosis requiring braces and surgery.

I think it is about time to recognize that the observation period is not helping people but on the contrary it hinders their proper treatment to stop a mild scoliosis from progressing to a severe scoliosis. It is time to change the 'OBSERVATION PERIOD"

Into an "ACTION PERIOD TO STOP THE MILD SCOLIOSIS FROM GETTING WORSE" with the 'ONE STITCH IN TIME TO SAVE NINE" approach, the .S.A.F.E. exercises.!

$$

$$$
$$$$$$$$$$$$$$$$$$$$$$$$$

7) THE REASON FOR A NEW CLASSIFICATION OF THE SO CALLED IDIOPATHIC SCOLIOSIS.

The reason I reclassified the idiopathic scoliosis to its possible causes is simple. In order to treat successfully a disease you have to know the cause, and by removing the cause, the treatments will be more effective and the patient will recover faster. The reason that many EXISTING treatments and exercises are not very successful in treating the so called idiopathic scoliosis is simple. They do not remove the cause of scoliosis. if you do not identify the cause of scoliosis and remove it , no matter what treatments or exercises the patient has, the cause will keep causing the abnormal curve to return and even get worse.

Take for example the positional infantile scoliosis with plagiocephaly. The only way that child will get better , both his scoliosis and malformed head is to _remove the cause first, in other words to change the position you hold the baby and the position that baby sleeps all the time, which caused the condition in the first place_. By just removing the cause and changing the position that the baby used to sleep, the child will get better ,even without any treatment . Just identify and remove the cause that's all needed. By removing the cause , the bad position the child was sleeping and with the proper exercises the child will get better faster. Some times when the doctors see a child with positional plagiocephaly, they tell the parents that the malformed head will correct itself , which is true most of the time. However when they fail to tell the parents to change the sleeping position of the baby , the plagiocephaly does not correct by itself and they have to use a custom-fit helmet to assist with changing the head's shape.

I read many books and watched some videos about correcting the scoliosis with exercising *balls, stretching here and stretching there, but I think with little success, because they say nothing about identifying and the removal of the cause. The patient pays for the treatments and does the exercises but because the cause is still there making the abnormal curve to get worse, no better. So in order to have good results with any treatment or exercises, first you have to identify the causative factor of the abnormal curve, remove the cause and then do the proper exercises and the scoliosis will stop from getting worse and <u>even reverse back to a straight , strong, healthy , dynamic and flexible spine!</u>*

So the main reason why the existing treatments are not very successful is that they do nothing to correct the cause of that scoliosis. It is like this, when there is a leaky roof and is causing damage to the ceiling below and you repair the ceiling without identifying the cause of the leak to fix it. You know that the ceiling will be damaged again, and again and it will be getting worse as long as the roof is leaking. The prudent thing to do is to identify the cause of the leak, fix the leak first and then fix the ceiling . That will be the end of the damage ceiling,
The same is true with scoliosis, unless you identify the cause of the abnormal curve and fix the cause first, no matter what you do to that curve it will

not be successful because the cause is still there causing the curve to get worse. It is as simple as that, but you have to identify and fix the cause first and by doing that the curve will reverse back to normal. It can only be three causes, a short leg, injury to the sacroiliac-lumbar area or bad postural habits.

If you are not sure check all three, starting with the mother of scoliosis, the lumbar-sacral-pelvis area.

8)THE SHAPE OF SCOLIOSIS

Most of the time the Scoliosis develops into two shapes

The idiopathic scoliosis usually has two shapes and most of the time starts at the low back at the Lunbosacral joints , the joints of the body, between the last lumbar vertebrae and the first sacral segment of the vertebral column and pelvis sacrum joints.

THE MOTHER OF SCOLIOSIS

I call this area, THE MOTHER OF ALL SCOLIOSIS, because that's where most of the abnormal curves of scoliosis occur.

a) One of the scoliosis' shape forms the English letter C

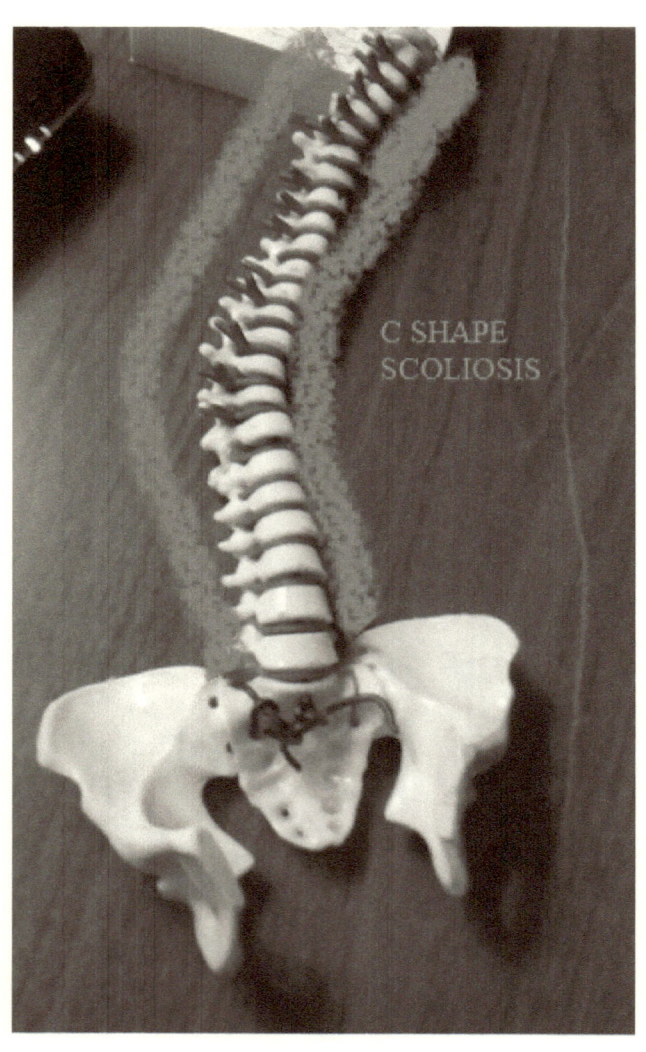

C SHAPE
SCOLIOSIS

and
b)the other shape of scoliosis is in the form of the
English letter S.

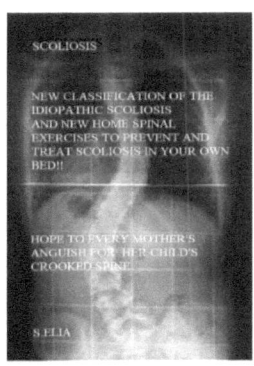

S SHAPE SCOLIOSIS DUE TO A SACROILIAC
PELVIS INJURY CAUSING A PRIMARY
LUMBAR CURVE AND A COMPENSATORY
SECONDARY CURVE IN THE THORACIC
SPINE   DUE TO THE RIGHTING REFLEX.

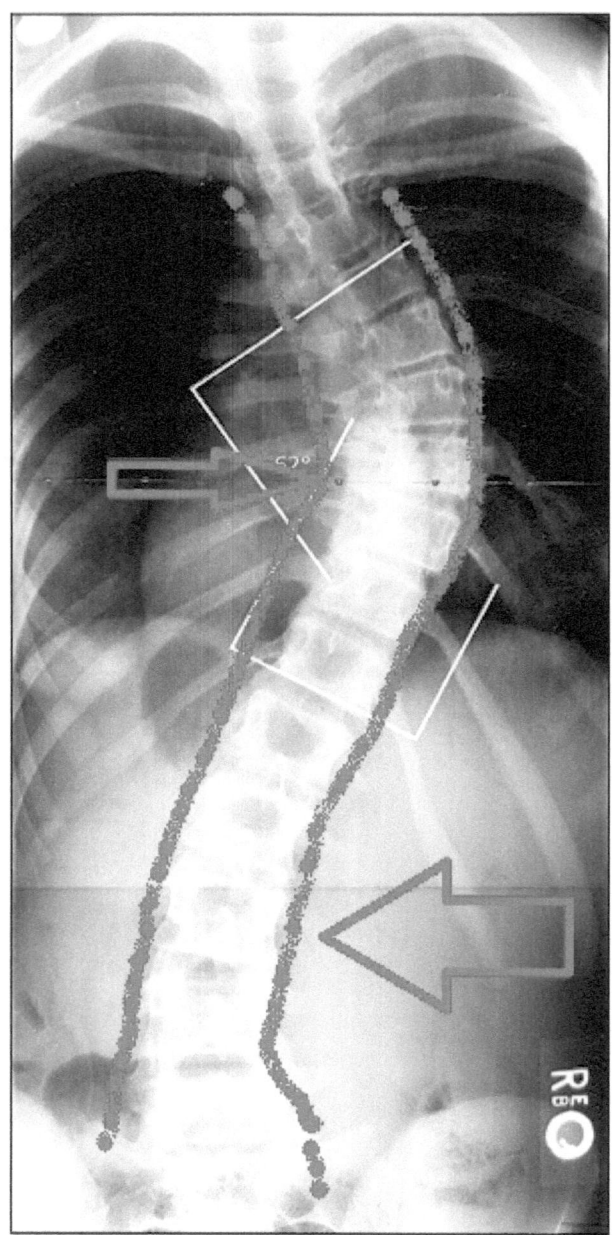

The idiopathic scoliosis usually starts any time after birth and with time the abnormal curve can progress to a severe incapacitating scoliosis causing many health problems.

Scoliosis is usually more prevalent in girls than the boys and the main reason for that, is the girls' motherhood instinct.

For years the scientific community and medical profession was baffled and still are, by this phenomenon and they wonder why such a discrepancy .

I have to admit that I had the same thinking and opinion for many years. You tend to believe and repeat of what you were taught , and what the books write until you learn otherwise, and you see the light at the end of the tunnel.

For years I was wondering why more girls had scoliosis than the boys, until One day while watching kids play in the neighborhood park, I had the AHA MOMENT .

Young kids mostly girls were lifting other younger kids and holding them on one side of their bodies and carrying them around . One of the girls was holding her back and she was limping a bit, after she lifted a heavy child and she carried the youngster around. She obviously had some pain and discomfort in her low back but she continued to play with the other kids after a short pause. After witnessing that, I figured out that if kids do this on a daily basis with their younger siblings, cousins, nephews etc that's HOW most of the kids get their scoliosis especially the girls with their motherly instinct.

 So I renamed the idiopathic scoliosis affecting the girls   "THE KIDS LIFTING BABIES SCOLIOSIS " OR BABYSITTING JUVENILE and adolescent SCOLIOSIS" When they baby-sit, PLAY or take care of babies. IN REALITY THIS IS A LIFTING INJURY TO THE LOW BACK, the sacroiliac joints and lumbar spine.
This might sound simple and the idiopathic scoliosis in girls , is not idiopathic anymore _but it has a serious cause that nobody paid any attention to it before._ Who could think that the idiopathic scoliosis is caused with kids lifting other kids while playing and having fun? We give girls dolls to play with and when they are older they like to play with LIVE HEAVY babies, siblingS, nieces, nephews or the neighbors' babies. Sometimes babies might be very heavy and if they have access to these kids daily for a long period of time AND THEY LIFT THEM AND CARRYING THEM AROUND   that's where their scoliosis start… BINGO!!!!!
Ever since that day that I saw the girls lifting other

kids, I saw other kids doing exactly the same thing, lifting heavy kids and carrying them around, usually short distances. In one particular occasion I saw a girl lifting   another younger girl, but heavy for her to lift, and she placed the younger girl on   her side straddling her pelvis and running around the playground trying to entertain the younger girl.

Now the girls want to have fun and entertain the younger kids but in the process they injure their backs and set themselves up for a life long suffering of low back injuries and the development of scoliosis. The girls do not know about the dangers of lifting heavy younger kids, and even their parents and their doctors do not know that, and that's the problem. The doctors never watch the kids play or what they do in their private lives, and they have no idea that kids are lifting heavy objects at that age. That's why they call it IDIOPATHIC SCOLIOSIS.

There is a need to educate the parents and everybody else including doctors why the girls and other youngsters are getting spinal injuries   and scoliosis from lifting heavy kids or other objects . That's the only way to stop or at least try to prevent this preventable condition called IDIOPATHIC SCOLIOSIS in girls and boys.

So the main reason why the girls have scoliosis more often than the boys, is the lifting of heavy kids and carrying them around. The motherhood instinct, and they pay the price for their effort to prepare for motherhood. They suffer from heavy lifting injuries to their low back which eventually leads to scoliosis.

And that is the simple explanation why girls have scoliosis more often than the boys do.

9)Other causes of scoliosis in girls and others .

1) bad postural habits, such as slouching on the sofa, sitting or standing, can cause scoliosis .
2) lifting heavy objects can cause strain in the low back and if untreated can lead to scoliosis.
3)carrying heavy objects such as schoolbags, handbags etc on one side of the body, eventually will cause scoliosis even in adults.
4)accidental falls and injury to the low back can cause scoliosis.
5) some form of gymnastic exercises, especially the spinal hyperextension, can cause injuries and even some fractures in the bones of the spine and can cause scoliosis.

6) exercises on a trampoline can lead to severe injuries, from falls and cause scoliosis , and even more catastrophic injuries to the spine. Always exercise with caution and under the supervision of expert professionals.

7) bad exercises , yes the wrong exercises can cause injuries to the spine and lead to scoliosis . Avoid any exercises of overextending or twisting the spine like the limbo dance.

8)Bad shoes with worn damaged heels on one or both shoes can cause strain in the low back and over time can cause scoliosis.

9)Tight clothing restricting the normal range of motion of the joints can cause strains to the knees, hip and low back and in rare cases can lead to scoliosis.

10) contact sports injuries, like hockey, football and wrestling can cause injuries leading to the development of scoliosis.

11) The wrong type of human hugs, the bear hugs, side hugs and violent unexpected hugs. Even when they hold the child in their arms and the child tries desperately to escape by twisting and turning his body violently can cause spinal injuries to the low back leading to scoliosis. I wrote about such injuries to kids in my book : the pros and cons of the human hug, by S.ELIA

published in EBook and paper back,, available amazon.com .

 12) A thick wallet or other objects on the back pockets of your trousers can cause imbalance on the sacrum -iliac joints when you sit down. The side where you keep your wallet pushes the pelvis on that side up causing a strain on the sacroiliac joint initiating the birth of scoliosis. Sometimes that strain can even cause a sciatica, sharp pain shooting down the leg. Some doctors call that form of sciatic pain, " the fat wallet syndrome". So keep your wallet and anything else for that matter, away from your back pocket.

From the above we can see that the injury to the spine can happen at any time and under different circumstances. The most common causes are heavy lifting, twisting at the waist while holding a heavy load, reaching and lifting, working in uncomfortable positions, standing or sitting in one position too long or a fall.

In other words , THE MOTHER of most causes of scoliosis is the injuries, sprains and strains on the pelvic joints, sacroiliac, hip, sacrum and L5. If these injuries are reported and treated early successfully the scoliosis will be avoided.

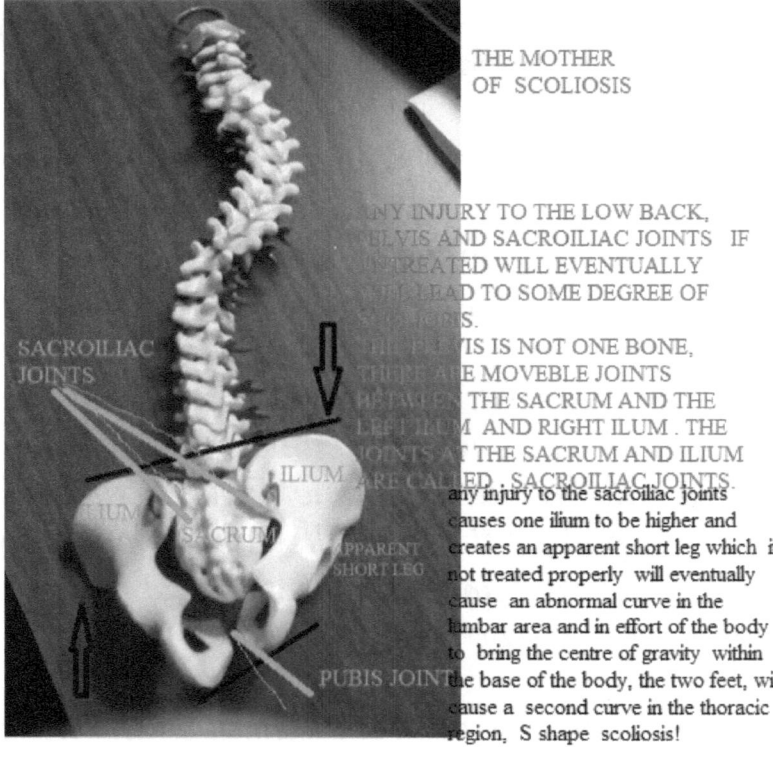

THE MOTHER
OF SCOLIOSIS

ANY INJURY TO THE LOW BACK, PELVIS AND SACROILIAC JOINTS IF UNTREATED WILL EVENTUALLY WILL LEAD TO SOME DEGREE OF SCOLIOSIS.
THE PELVIS IS NOT ONE BONE, THERE ARE MOVEBLE JOINTS BETWEEN THE SACRUM AND THE LEFT ILIUM AND RIGHT ILUM . THE JOINTS AT THE SACRUM AND ILIUM ARE CALLED , SACROILIAC JOINTS. any injury to the sacroiliac joints causes one ilium to be higher and creates an apparent short leg which if not treated properly will eventually cause an abnormal curve in the lumbar area and in effort of the body to bring the centre of gravity within the base of the body, the two feet, will cause a second curve in the thoracic region, S shape scoliosis!

SACROILIAC JOINTS

ILIUM

SACRUM

APPARENT SHORT LEG

PUBIS JOINT

In a nutshell that's how scoliosis develops over time.
You can take precautions to prevent such injuries and avoid the possibility of having scoliosis. However no matter what precautions you take accidents do happen when you least expect it, even when you just bend over to pick up a pencil. In such cases the early diagnosis and treatment is necessary to avoid long debilitating conditions such as scoliosis and eventually osteoarthritis changes in the damaged joints.

The good news is that with the proper exercises you can train your spine, like most athletes do and have a strong , healthy and flexible spine which can prevent injuries to the low back that eventually cause scoliosis.

Even if you have some strain in your sacroiliac joints and low back with an elastic support for your sacroiliac joints in the acute phase, and the SPINAL ACTIVE FLEXION EXERCISES, you will have a good chance to recover completely and avoid scoliosis.

10)HOW TO PREVENT low back injuries and SCOLIOSIS

There is a saying that "an once of prevention is worth a ton of   therapy."

The best way to prevent scoliosis is exercise , the right exercises that prevents what causes scoliosis which can start as early as soon as a child is born.

By Exercising and avoiding what causes injuries to the joints of your spine and especially the sacroiliac- pelvic joints which is the base and support of the spine , you can prevent low back injuries and scoliosis.

Below is a list of what can cause injuries and scoliosis of the spine. Read and memorized this list and especially learn How to protect your low back from injury that might lead to scoliosis in your every day life.

1) DO NOT SLEEP ON YOUR STOMACH.
Sleeping on your stomach causes strain to your neck and low back and can be the beginning of scoliosis. The best way to sleep is face up and on your side with a small pillow to rest your head on, but not always sleeping on the same side. Sleeping on just one side causes scoliosis and plagiocephaly in kids.
2) DO NOT PLAY ON THE TRAMPOLINE.
you can hurt your back and other parts of your body , from an accidental fall thus creating the chance of developing scoliosis
3)NO HEAVY LIFTING AND ALWAYS BEND YOUR KNEES
When you have to lift anything , even a pencil. Proper precautions on how to lift and good postural habits are essential for all people whether they have scoliosis or a straight spine, to protect their spine from injury.

4)) DO NOT CARRY HEAVY OBJECTS OR OVERLOADED backpacks and never carry any objects on one side of your body, because that forces your spine into a scoliosis curve and over time it might cause scoliosis.

5) AVOID BAD SITTING POSITIONS ,

When you read , work on the computer, at the table, at school and especially when you watch television or movies. Bad sitting positions put a lot of strain on the sacral -pelvis area and can cause a lot of health problems including scoliosis and other postural problems.

6)IF YOU HAVE YOUNGER SIBLINGS OR NIECES

and nephews do not lift them and never hold them on one side of your body , as this has the potential to cause strain on your back and eventually scoliosis.

If you baby-sit younger kids or babies never lift them, that's   how most of the girls get their scoliosis.

7)   Avoid practical jokes and horsing around. Many people had scoliosis and even catastrophic injuries from such practical jokes.

8) AVOID   CONTACT SPORTS   like football, wrestling, and hockey. Many people had lifelong severe injuries to their spine including scoliosis from such sports.

9)AVOID EXCESSIVE HUGGING , Especially when your body is in an awkward position and definitely you should Avoid sideways hugs and violent hugs like the " bear hug."

10)if you have to do heavy lifting or work in the garden or anything that has to do with a lot of bending and lifting, use an elastic brace to protect your back. Do as the athletes of heavy lifting do to protect their spines from lifting weights injuries, they use a protective low back belt.

11) if you have pain from strain or sprain in your low back do not ignore it. Use an elastic brace to protect your spine from further injury. If the pain does not go away in a few days see your doctor . By treating an injury early you prevent it from becoming chronic and cause other health problems including scoliosis.

12) EXERCISE, the last but the most important of all, is to exercise. Exercises are good for any age even for babies. I saw a pediatrician on television giving the mother of a child a prescription… for more exercises for her child. And that's good news. More doctors should give such prescriptions. The right exercises will make the spine strong, healthy and flexible and when you have strong healthy spinal muscles will protect the spine from any injuries. That's why I designed the SPINAL ACTIVE FLEXION

EXERCISES in short S.A.F.E.
These exercise are good   for prevention of
scoliosis by making the spinal muscles strong and
the spine healthy and flexible.
These exercises are also very good at correcting
any misalignments in the pelvis and spinal joint
thus stopping the progression of any abnormal
curves in the spine and even reversing it back to
normal. There will be detailed description with
pictures of these exercises later on in this book
under the heading : prevention and treatment of
scoliosis.

These exercises are designed to make your spine
strong, healthy and more flexible and in the
process to correct any abnormal curves of the spine
such as scoliosis, kyphosis and lordosis. you do not
need any exercise balls or to push your spine one
way or another. these exercises will correct any
curve of the spine by making your spinal muscles
strong on both sides of the spine plus will correct
any misalignment of the pelvic joints which usually
is the mother (the cause) of the scoliosis.... but you
have to do them daily every day for ever.. or at
least when your scoliosis is gone.

11)SIGNS AND SYMPTOMS OF SCOLIOSIS

People with scoliosis might have pain in the low back, neck and shoulder blades and sometimes in the early stages, the scoliosis can be without pain.

When the scoliosis is severe with the spine severely crooked it can cause serious health problems affecting the lungs, heart and other the parts of the body .

People with scoliosis have uneven shoulders, one shoulder blade is more prominent than the other, and have a rib hump One hip higher than the other uneven hips arms or leg lengths.

Sometimes other people, family friends and classmates notice the scoliosis first, for the obvious reason that people with scoliosis they cannot see their spine on their back, but others have a better view of others' spine.

12) DIAGNOSIS OF SCOLIOSIS

Anybody can see a crooked spine when the abnormal curve is severe , but a definite diagnosis is made by taking a

full x ray   of the spine with the patient standing, AP   and lateral views and measuring the COBB angle to see how bad the abnormal curve is.
The greater the   COBB angle the worse the scoliosis is .

There is also a simple test the" ADAMS TEST"
that anybody can perform at home, by asking the
patient to bend forward with the knees straight and
observing the spine to see if the spine is straight
or if there is an abnormality on   one side of the
spine(the curve of the scoliosis) a rib hump   where
the ribs on one side protrude. If the spine is
straight when the patient bend forward, the test is
negative and there is no scoliosis present. If the
spine is not straight and has obvious sideways
curves , the spine has scoliosis and further
investigations and x-rays are necessary to see if
there is any pathology present or IF it is just an
abnormal curve with a measurable COBB angle.
If there is pain present when the patient bends
over, it means that there is a problem in the spine
and should be investigated by a doctor and if
necessary to take an x-ray for proper diagnosis
and treatment .

If there is scoliosis but no pathology present, you
try to determine what is causing that abnormal
curve, so that the proper treatment is more effective
when you eliminate that cause.

As we described the causes of scoliosis above in the re-classification of the idiopathic scoliosis, when the child is 0-3 years we will be looking as the causes of the scoliosis :

a) positional infantile scoliosis with positional plagiocephaly , the way they hold the baby, and what position the baby sleeps .

and *b) the traumatic infantile scoliosis,* any accidental falls.

For the ages of 3 -20 years of age we will be looking for the causes of

1) the bad habits or postural juvenile and adolescent scoliosis in which the kids have bad slouching habits when the sit, stand, watch television or play video games.

2) the causes of the baby-sitting juvenile and adolescent scoliosis which is the access to other kids , baby-sitting, playing and lifting other heavy kids.

3) the causes of the traumatic juvenile and adolescent scoliosis which are the accidental falls, lifting heavy objects , or carrying heavy objects such as school bags on one side of their bodies causing sprains and strains at the lower back.

4) check for a true short leg by measuring the legs. If there is a true short leg present you have to *correct it by a heel lift or a shoe lift. that's the only way to have good results with any treatment!*

13)Eliminate the causes of scoliosis to have better results with the treatment.

When the diagnosis is made and we know what is causing that abnormal spinal curve, the first thing to do is eliminate that cause so that the treatments are effective.

The x-rays will show if there is a fracture, or any pathology in the bones of the spine, where the scoliosis start, any misalignment of the vertebrae , the pelvis and what shape the scoliosis is. A shape C or an S shape.

If the x-rays do not show any pathology and no scoliosis is present, that's very good news. The spine is healthy and no reason to worry but it is a good opportunity to take preventative measures to keep the spine healthy , strong and flexible with the right exercises..

*IF THERE IS SCOLIOSIS, The shape of scoliosis
and the age of the patient will give clues if it is
postural with a C shape or an S shape which
indicates that it started in the low back, pelvis area
due to a strain or sprain in the sacroiliac joints
from lifting heavy objects heavy babies in girls
scoliosis, or due to an apparent or a true short leg.*

*When we identify that there is an abnormal spinal
curve, called scoliosis and we identify the possible
cause of that scoliosis, first we make sure to
remove that cause and with the spinal active
flexion exercises, in short S.A.F.E. the patient
will have a good chance to stop the progression of
that abnormal curve and even reverse back to
normal.*

14)THE S.A.F.E. EXERCISES.

After many years of studying, researching and observing human spines both normal and abnormal with scoliosis, kyphosis and lordosis, I came to the conclusion that the best way to prevent and treat the abnormal curves of the spine is the right exercises and the S.A.F.E. exercises if done daily in the privacy of your home , even in your own bed, can do that.

Why are the exercises s.a.f.e   the best exercises to prevent and treat scoliosis?. Because the s.a.f.e exercises are based on the   Adam's test which tells us that flexing the spine over and over again will strengthen the muscles of the spine and in the process to straighten the spine as well. These exercises are also designed to correct the root cause where the scoliosis starts at the base of the spine the sacroiliac joints and all pelvic joints which are the mother of most scoliosis.

These exercises are also based on years of observations how the top athletes are trained and what exercises they do to have a strong , healthy and flexible spine. These athletes almost never have any scoliosis .

I designed these exercises for the purpose of correcting the root cause of scoliosis, which is the misalignment of the lumbar spinal bones, the sacrum and the pelvic bones called ilium one on each side of the sacrum.

LUMBAR 5
VERTEBRA

SACROILIAC
JOINTS

LUMBAR 5
VERTEBRA

RIGHT ILIUM

LEFT ILIUM

SACRUM

THE AREA WHERE   THE CAUSE OF SCOLIOSIS MOST OF THE TIME START

But in order to get the best results with these exercises you have to eliminate what is causing the scoliosis first. Without eliminating the cause of scoliosis, no treatment or exercises can be successful.

Exercise with the s.a.fe. Exercises at least twice daily on   an empty stomach.

15)How to check your kids spine to see if there is scoliosis present.

 The parents are in a good position to check their kids if they have scoliosis or not, because they see them every day and they will notice any changes to their child, the way they stand, walk or sit.
When the child is still a baby you can check when you change or dress the baby. Look at their spine to see if it looks straight and put the child on your knees and run your index   and middle finger along the spine of the child to see if it s straight or has any abnormality. If you notice any abnormality to the spine or the face and head, check with the doctor to make the diagnosis and recommend the proper treatment. If the child has positional plagiocephaly, a condition that disfigures   the head of the baby when it sleeps on one side all the time, you have to change the position that the baby sleeps and the baby's head will return to normal.

It is also good to exercise the baby every time you change it with mild knee to chest exercises. let the baby move freely the feet and hands for a while. When the child is over 3 years old you can check the child's spine by just asking the child to bend over and you watch their spine to see if it is straight or has any abnormal curves along the spine. This is the Adam's test that all doctors perform to see if there are any indications of an abnormal curve of the spine. When you perform this test the spine should be exposed. For the girls you can ask them to put on their shirt backwards . If you notice any abnormality, check with your family doctor for proper diagnosis and any treatments if needed. Early detection is easier to stop the progression of the abnormal curve and even reverse it. The so called " A stitch on time saves nine." the S.A.F.E. exercises.

As a parent you have the chance to observe your child all the time and especially during the summer time , at the beach or in the backyard and if you see any changes in their appearances , check them with the Adam's test to make sure that there is no scoliosis present. Any time you are not sure ask your doctor to check it out. That's why there are doctors.

16) EXISTING TREATMENTS FOR SCOLIOSIS

There are many treatments for scoliosis. Some of them are good some of them so-so and some risky , like the corrective surgery with fusion and the use of rods in the spine. Although, I must say that surgery in many cases is absolutely necessary and most of the time with good results . Most children when they are first diagnosed with a mild scoliosis they are told to wait and see, the observation period, how the curve will develop in six months to a year without any treatments or advice. And that's the biggest mistake and the waste of valuable time.

The National Institute of Arthritis and Musculoskeletal Diseases recommends these three treatments:
1) Observation: When a curve is detected early on in a growing child, most doctors are likely to recommend regular check-ups and observe the scoliosis without any intervention. that's why is called observation period, they just observe without any treatment.

2)Bracing: If the curve is moderate and your child is still growing, braces may be recommended.

These will be fitted according to the curve of the spine and will be regularly monitored by the doctor.

3)Surgery: If the severity of the curve is increasing and your child is still growing, surgery may be recommended.

And the last one
  4)which of course   is the conservative treatments with exercises and different modalities such as traction, exercise balls etc.

Lets examine each recommendation separately and see if those recommendations are adequate, .
1) the observation period.
 I think that's the biggest mistake for not treating scoliosis immediately while the curve is small and easy to manage. It is a missed opportunity to treat and stop the progression of the abnormal curve called scoliosis before it becomes a severe scoliosis requiring heavy braces and surgery.

  To   "the wait and see approach " or the so called observation period, I have to agree with the view of Dr. 'John H. Moe .

   Dr. 'John H. Moe 1905-1988   was a University of Minnesota orthopedic surgeon, who

*founded the Scoliosis Research Society in 1966
and he began a "do not delay" campaign for
scoliosis, and he wrote "procrastination was
the most pernicious problem in idiopathic
scoliosis and sad to see a child come with a
severe curve requiring surgery with X-rays taken
many years before showing a mild curve that
could have been easily treated with a brace.
46'Dangerous Curve" campaign .*

*When the abnormal curve gets worse in six
months or a year they advice them to use a
brace for a period of time and if that does not
help the scoliosis they have surgery to fuse the
spine and use rods to straighten the spine.*
Millions of people are diagnosed with mild
scoliosis every year and with the existing protocol
of treating scoliosis, especially the "WAIT AND
SEE APPROACH" or the so called
"OBSERVATION PERIOD" their scoliosis will
progress to severe scoliosis requiring braces and
surgery.
I think it is about time to recognize that the
observation period is not helping people but on the
contrary it hinders their proper treatment to stop a
mild scoliosis from progressing to a severe
scoliosis.
It is time to change the 'OBSERVATION
PERIOD"

Into an "ACTION PERIOD TO STOP THE MILD SCOLIOSIS FROM GETTING WORSE" with the 'ONE STITCH IN TIME TO SAVE NINE" approach, the .S.A.F.E. exercises.!
The best time to stop the progression of scoliosis and even reverse it is when the abnormal curve is still small and easier to manage.

With the "one stitch in time to save nine", you find the cause of that abnormal curve, which is either postural, from bad postural habits, traumatic to the low back, pelvic sacral joints, or a true short leg. You correct the causative factor and with the spinal active exercises, S.A.F.E., you will have better chance in stopping the progression and reversing scoliosis.

That's where you have to start treating the abnormal curve, when it is still small and manageable, and not to waste any valuable time observing a small scoliosis to become severe, requiring surgery fusion and rods in the spine.

2) Bracing : the use of spinal braces trying to stop the progression of the curve and even reverse the abnormal spinal curve.

The basic idea of bracing is good and it will have better results if it was initiated when the scoliosis was first diagnosed along with corrective spinal exercises to make the spine stronger, healthy and flexible.

The idea of bracing is not new. It has been used from time immemorial for preventing and treating human ailments, such as low back injuries and other joint injuries.

At one time it was fashionable for women to wear body elastic or fabric garments similar to today's braces called corset, to hold their posture in good shape.

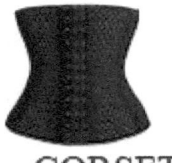

CORSET

A corset is a garment worn under the clothes, to hold and train the upper body into a desired shape, a smaller waist or larger bottom, for aesthetic purposes and to improve their posture. I think that the fashionable corset was protecting women from any abnormal curves of the spine, as they were constantly trying to improve their posture . That it was also preventing them from bad postural habits and protecting their low back from any injury when they were lifting something heavy . And that was good for them and a terrific idea.

The use of a brace to treat scoliosis, at least

prevents people from slouching and bad postural positions and that has an effect in stopping the progression of scoliosis. I t is also protecting the low back from further injury when they lift something, the so called lifting accidents. When you combine bracing with the right exercises, preferably the S.A.F.E. exercises, the ones I designed to correct any misalignments in the lumbar-sacral area, it will be easier to stop the progression and even reverse it back to a normal position.

The idea of bracing sounds good, but a prolong use of any brace is not a good idea as it causes the muscles to become spastic and eventually weak . On the other side, exercises promote healing, strength and flexibility of the spine.

The use of a brace is essential in treating any injury to the spine or any other joint of the body in the acute phase of an injury. The brace stabilizes , supports and protects the injured low back or any other joints of the body until that injury is healed properly.

The use of a supportive brace is a good idea anytime you do heavy lifting to protect the spine from any injury, sprain or strain. The weight lifters and others are using some sort of brace to protect their spines from any injury while they lift heavy weights.

However people should avoid prolong use of any brace or a corset, as the joints become stiff and the muscles weak and wasted from disuse. Use a brace only in the acute injury state or when you do some heavy work and exercise regularly to have strong muscles and healthy flexible joints.

3)Surgery: If the severity of the curve is increasing and your child is still growing, surgery may be recommended.

Sometimes the abnormal spinal curve keeps growing until it becomes so severe that causes health problems such as deformity of the chest with breathing problems, heart lung problems, pain and deformity of the spine which can affect many functions of the body due to the involvement of the spinal cord and spinal nerves.

So when the abnormal spinal curve becomes severe and causes health problems, it is necessary for surgery of the spine, to fuse some vertebrae(spinal bones) and insert rods to hold the spine in a straight position. Spinal surgery has potentially major health risks but sometimes it is absolutely necessary. As time goes buy the spinal surgeons improve their surgical techniques and skills and most of the time the spinal surgeries are successful. However the patients loose the flexibility of their spine. But if you loose some

flexibility and avoid a lot of health problems, I think it is a good trade!
Now if there is a way to reverse that scoliosis before it becomes so severe requiring surgical intervention it is even better for the patients and their families !!!

4)the conservative treatments.

There are many conservative treatments for scoliosis. Some of them are good , some of them fair some of them are risky. There are physiotherapy exercises, yoga exercises, Pilates exercises, Schroth scoliosis treatment and others but I do not know how effective are in treating scoliosis. I read some comments from some of the curvy girls that they tried those conservative treatments, but they ended up having surgery at the end. So I figured out that those treatments were not able to stop the progression of their scoliosis. Some of those exercises and treatments are good and are supposed to help those with scoliosis., My guess is that those who supervised and teach those treatments or exercises, failed to identify the cause of scoliosis and When you do not identify the cause and remove it, no treatment or exercise can be successful in stopping the progression of scoliosis.
The same thing can be said about the various modalities that use to treat scoliosis. The spinal

tractions, the inverted traction, exercising balls, various chairs that are supposed to correct the scoliosis will not be effective unless you find what is causing that abnormal curve and remove that cause first. If the cause that initiate the scoliosis is still there, it will keep making the scoliosis worse, no matter what modality or anything else you use. If the patient has a true short leg that is causing the primary and secondary spinal curves of scoliosis , unless you fix that short leg first with a heel-lift or a shoe lift, you will never be able to correct that scoliosis no matter how many exercises or other treatments that patient has. It is as simple as that, first find the cause, remove it and then treat or exercise to correct the scoliosis and especially in the early stage of scoliosis when it is diagnosed first and the curve was still small. The same can be said when the scoliosis is caused by bad postural habits, slouching when sitting , watching television etc . No matter how many exercises or treatments the patient has, if after the treatments or exercises goes back to slouching , the treatments and exercises will do nothing for the patients until they eliminate their bad postural habits.

When you identify the cause, remove it and then do the exercises and the treatments, the scoliosis will stop from getting worse and even reverse back to normal.

To summarize it , any treatment or exercise will be effective only after you identify ,remove and eliminate the cause of that abnormal curve called scoliosis. Without identifying the cause and removing the cause of that scoliosis, it will be a waste of time and money while the curve will keep growing until it requires surgical correction.

All the treatments with exercises or modalities are classified as conservative treatments.
The spinal active flexion exercises , S.A.FE. which I designed are considered conservative treatments for the prevention and treatment of the so called idiopathic scoliosis.
After many years of studying, researching and observing human spines both normal and abnormal with scoliosis, kyphosis and lordosis, I came to the conclusion that the best way to prevent and treat the abnormal curves of the spine is the proper exercises and the S.A.F.E. if done daily in the privacy of your home , even in your own bed, can do that.

These exercises are the best for the prevention and correction of any spinal curves, scoliosis, kyphosis and lordosis by making the spinal muscles stronger and the spine healthier, stronger and more flexible

In 1865 William ADAMS was the first to describe

" the forward bending test " for scoliosis, and all doctors use this test to diagnose the functional or structural scoliosis.

William Adams made a very good observation about the abnormal curve of the spine called scoliosis but nobody else added anything to that observation or took advantage of that observation up to now.

Based on Williams Adams observation and years of observation how athletes train and exercise to have a strong, healthy, flexible spine without any abnormal curves or scoliosis, I designed specific exercises for the spine so that by bending and exercising the spine for long periods of time, while lying face up to avoid the gravity factor, it will make the muscles strong and the spine stronger , flexible and keep it almost straight.

With the spinal active flexion exercises S.A.F.E. , will also help the re-alignment of their pelvic and hip joints to restore normal function to those joints. These joints is the mother of any scoliosis starting in that area and by correcting these pelvic joints it will restore normal function of those joints and a straight spine without scoliosis.

And that's the main purpose of the s.a.f.e. exercises to prevent and treat the scoliosis that starts at the lumbar-sacral joints which is the base of the spine..

17)The birth of the s.a.f.e. exercises for the prevention and treatment of the so called

idiopathic scoliosis.

After many years of studying, researching and observing human spines both normal and abnormal with scoliosis, kyphosis and lordosis, I came to the conclusion that people can injure their spine at any time by just bending down the wrong way to pick up a pencil, or slouching on their favorite sofa watching television or just lifting and carrying a small object. I tried to fix injured and crooked spines by using taping, bracing, traction, manipulation, electrotherapy and exercises. I even used the principle of the exercising ball trying to push the crooked spine back to straight. I found out that this method is not effective to straighten out the scoliosis curve unless you fix the cause of that curve first. A spinal surgeon explaining spinal surgery, put it this way. "You can push that curve back to straight but it does not stay straight, it keeps going back to an abnormal curve and that's why there is a need for the supporting rods".

Finally after many years of trying to correct the spinal curves, I came to the conclusion that the best way to prevent and treat the abnormal curves of the spine is the right spinal exercises and the patient has to do the exercises daily. Exercises is the key for prevention and treatment of scoliosis by making the spine , strong, healthy and flexible. I think that the spinal active flexion exercises , in short S.A.F.E. that I designed, are the best exercise for prevention and treatment of the so called idiopathic scoliosis. when I was looking for the best exercises to prevent and treat scoliosis, I took into account the normal range of the spinal motion, flexion ,less extension and even less rotation and the exercises that have the potential to correct any misalignments in the spine.

The bending forwards Adam's test gave me the clue and the answer. Every time the bending forwards Adam's test is performed the spine tries to straighten. When there is a functional scoliosis the curve disappears and in structural scoliosis the abnormal curve tries to straighten out too. So I figured out that if someone with scoliosis does flexion exercises, over and over again on a daily basis, with time the spine will straighten and return to its normal shape. I also spend a lot of time observing the exercising habits of people that have strong flexible spines without any abnormal curves, like the professional athletes that exercises daily. The body builders, the swimmers, the weight lifters and others. When I combined the Adam's forwards test ,with some of the exercises or variation of those exercises, that professional athletes do, and the exercises that have the potential to correct

any misaligned pelvic-sacral-
lumbar joints, the spinal active
flexion exercises in short
S.A.F.E. were (born)developed.
These exercises are the best in
stopping the progression of the
scoliosis and even reversing the
abnormal curve, but you have to
remove or correct the cause of
that curve first.

Since idiopathic scoliosis means
that it has no known cause, I
looked closely for that elusive
cause. Just because they named the
scoliosis idiopathic with that
archaic name, it does not mean
that it has no cause. it just
means that there is no obvious
cause yet. Besides if the child
was born with a normal spine and
then it developed an abnormal
curve it must have a cause for
that curve to develop. Something
caused that curve to develop and
there is always a cause for that
curve, an injury or a postural
position.
During my quest for that unknown
cause of the idiopathic

scoliosis, I found that there are many obvious causes, not just one, depending on the age of the individual with scoliosis. So I re-classified the idiopathic scoliosis according to the age of the patient and the cause of that curve which I list in this book. Although there are several causes, in reality there are only three major causes and a variation of the three causes, depending on the age of the individual , from the time of infancy to adulthood.

The most common cause of the idiopathic scoliosis is a lifting and twisting injury to the low back, creating an imbalance at the base of the spine, the pelvis-sacrum-lumbar area. That imbalance creates an apparent short leg and a primary curve to the lumbar-sacral area and if left untreated will cause a secondary curve in the thoracic spine due to the righting reflex of the body.

The righting reflex, is a reflex that

corrects the orientation of the body when
it is taken out of its normal upright
position.

In other words the body tries to
bring the centre of gravity
within its base, which for the
human body is the two feet.
This type of injury can occur at
any age from infancy to
adulthood and believe it
or not is more prevalent to
girls(the baby-sitting adolescent
scoliosis) due to their motherhood
instinct, when they pretend to be
the mothers of younger heavy kids
by lifting and carrying them
around.
The second most common cause of
idiopathic scoliosis is due to
bad postural habits, slouching,
prolong sitting the wrong way at
home , school, playing video
games, when they watch
television etc. since this type
of scoliosis is caused by bad
postural habits is called
postural scoliosis according to
the patients age, this type of

scoliosis can be a C shape or an S shape.

 The least common type of scoliosis is when the patient has a true short leg, one leg is shorter than the other. The short leg causes an imbalance to the pelvis-sacrum- lumbar area, creating an abnormal primary curve in the lumbar area(low back) and if left untreated will create a secondary curve in the thoracic spine, again due to the righting reflex of the body.

The obvious treatment for the true short leg is to correct the length of the short leg
and spinal exercises preferable the S.A,F.E.. exercises to mobilize and correct the sacral-pelvis area.

The best time to treat scoliosis is when the spinal curve is till small and easier to treat and correct. The "stitch in time to save nine" as the wise proverb says.

It is my opinion that the 'wait and see approach' or the so called "observation period " should be replaced immediately with "the action period to correct and reverse " the abnormal curve called scoliosis. I see no reason why delay and waste precious time with the so called "observation period", which does not serve the needs of the patients. If that observation period is used properly can save a lot of patients from getting worse, requiring bracing and surgery.

The s.a.f.e. exercises are good for preventing scoliosis by making the spinal muscles stronger and the spine strong and more flexible safeguarding it from an injury.

The s.a.f.e. exercises are good at stopping the progression of the abnormal curve ,by correcting any imbalance to the lumbar-sacral-pelvic area promoting healing and early rehabilitation.
The S.A.F.E. exercises are designed specifically according to

the normal motions of the spine
to increase the normal range of
motion and in the process to make
it more flexible, stronger and
bring back the normal range of
motion to any joints that were
restricted by the abnormal curve.

Many international athletes do
similar exercises or variation of
the s.a.f.e. exercises to train
for a strong, flexible and healthy
spine without any abnormal curves.
Their postures are perfect without
any abnormal curves and it is the
envy of many.

William Adams made that famous
observation that every scoliosis
when is flexed(bend) forwards
tries to straighten up. It is like
the spine is trying to (tell us)
show us the way to correct that
abnormal curve.
That is exactly what I did. I
designed specific exercises to
flex the spine, over and over
again until the abnormal curve is
stopped, or eliminated. I even

removed the gravity factor which
is present when the patient is
standing and I designed the
spinal exercises to do the
exercises lying down face up.

The S.A.F.E exercises are easy to
do in the privacy of your home ,
even in your own bed without any
equipment. No need to buy
expensive equipment or wasting
traveling time to the gym and
paying membership fees.

These exercises are good for
anyone that has a spine and I hope
many people will seize the
opportunity to start exercising
with these exercise to prevent
scoliosis by making their spines
stronger , flexible and healthier.

However these exercises are not
indented for people that have
fractures, pathology or spinal
surgery and rods in their spines!
If that is your case, consult
your doctor for proper diagnosis,

treatments and suitable exercises.

It is my hope that all people affected with scoliosis, kyphosis and lordosis will greatly benefit by exercising with these exercise daily.

18)Prevention and correction of scoliosis with the spinal active flexion exercises in short S.A.F.E.

You can do these exercises in the privacy of your own home without any equipment, exercising balls or anything else.
You can do the exercises on a mat or even in your own bed.

You do these exercises at least twice a day morning and evening and always on an EMPTY STOMACH, and never after you had a meal.
The exercises are easy to do and you go easy at the beginning and never strain yourself.
Have a routine exercising time and keep a diary with photos of the improvement achieved for motivation and encouragement.

If you have friends or know other people with scoliosis form a group and do the exercises together at least once or twice a month or sooner if you want, for support and encouragement.

N.B. These exercises are good for anybody that has a spine, but not intended for people with spinal fractures, pathology or had surgery and spinal fusion with rod in their spines. If that's your case, consult your doctor for advise before doing any exercises

And here are the corrective spinal active flexion exercises S.A.F.E. in short.

*19)THE SPINAL ACTIVE FLEXION
EXERCISES(S.A.F.E.)*

Basic precaution and instructions.

**N.B. You do these exercises on an empty stomach
and never after a meal or a big drink.**

***YOU ALWAYS TAKE IT EASY AND NEVER
STRAIN YOURSELF.***

**If any exercise causes pain , skip it and do
another exercise until you are stronger and more
flexible**

**Avoid any spinal extension exercises. With the
scoliosis the bones of the spine are crowded
twisted and jammed and any extension exercises**

aggravates the crowding bones making the scoliosis worse!!

##
###########

.

 DESCRIPTIONS OF THE   HOME S.A.F.E. EXERCISES .
  HERE ARE THE   HOME EXERCISES WHICH I DESIGNED AND I CALL S.A.F.E. (SPINAL ACTIVE FLEXION EXERCISES)

EXERCISE ONE.

 Lie face up on a mat or a mattress ,
Interlock your fingers and place them under your head.

LIE FACE UP
ON A MAT OR
A MATRESS

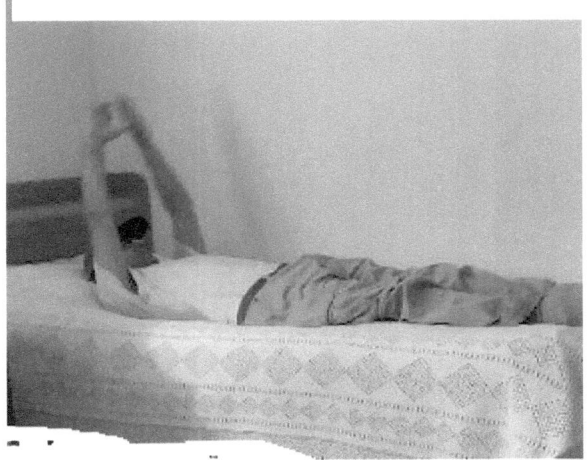

INTERLOCK
YOUR FINGERS
AND PLACE
THEM UNDER
YOUR HEAD

Take a deep breath in expanding your chest as much as possible.
Exhale slowly. Repeat 5 times.

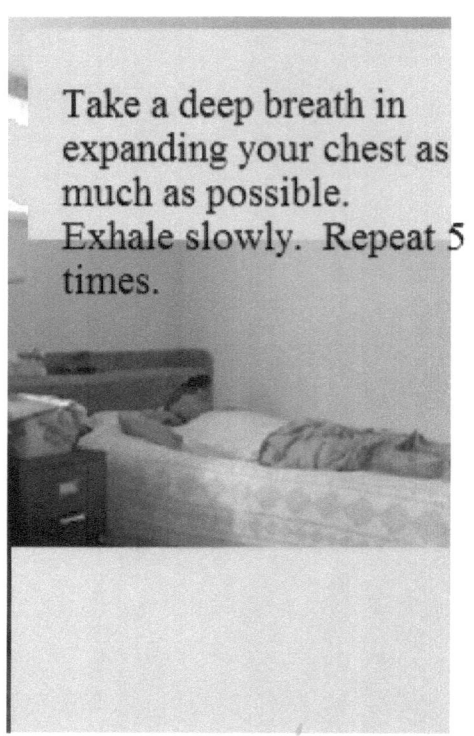

Take a deep breath in expanding your chest as much as possible.
Exhale slowly. Repeat 5 times.

This exercise is good for expanding your chest cavity stretching your ribs and your shoulder blades.. it will exercise and strengthen the chest muscles and will restore normal range of motion to the ribs reducing any rib hump

@@@@@@@@@@@@@@@@@@@@@@@
@@@@@@@

Exercise two
Lying face up with your hands
interlocked under your head

Then bring your bent elbows towards your nose as
far as you can

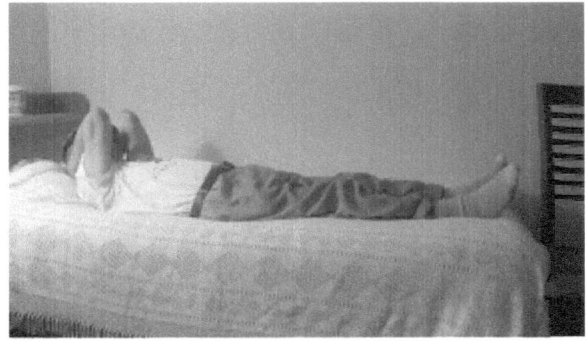

And then back towards the mattress pressing on the
mattress.

lying face up,
interlock fingers
and place them
under your head

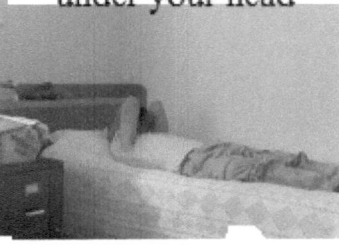

bring your elbows
towards your face ,
then back pressing on
the mattress

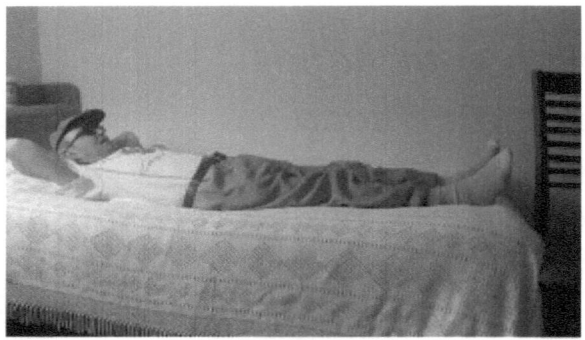

Repeat this motion of your elbows towards your nose and back to pressing on the mattress 10-20 times.

Do not overdo it but keep increasing the repetitions as you get stronger.

These exercises are the best for strengthening your upper chest and shoulder muscles and mobilizing your upper thoracic and cervical spine.

@@@@@@@@@@@@@@@@@@@@@@@@@
@@@@@@@

Rest   by taking   deep breaths   expanding your chest as much as possible and exhaling slowly.

@@@@@@@@@@@@@@@@@@@@@@@@@
@@@@@@@

EXERCISE THREE

From the same position, face up, hands interlocked behind the head
Bend your right knee and let it down   on the mattress
* and raise your head towards the chest   as far as you can without straining yourself.*
* Repeat 5 times and keep increasing them as you get stronger. Never over do it .*

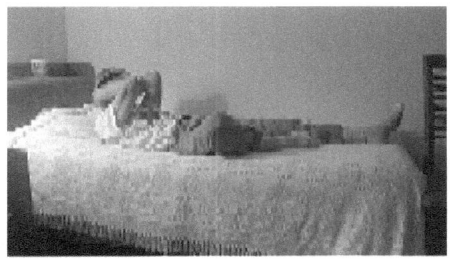

Repeat the same exercise with your left knee
Bend your left knee ,
Let it down on you left side
and raise the head towards your chest five times

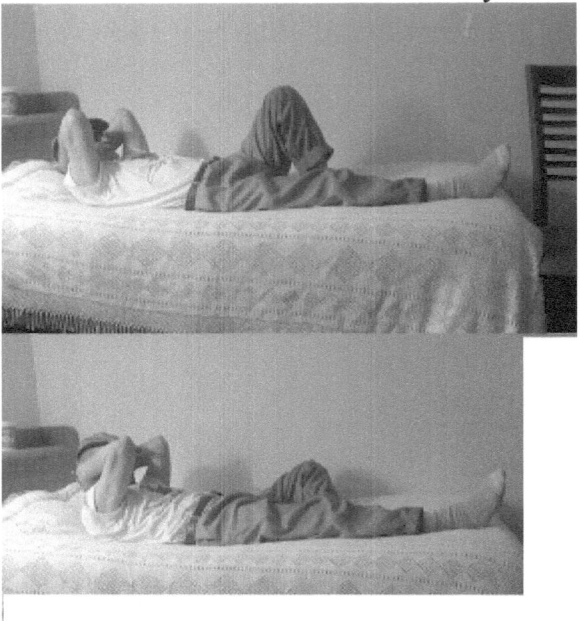

Repeat this exercise 5 times and as you get stronger and more flexible you increase the repetitions.

N.B. This is not a sit up exercise and do not try to sit up, you just raise your head towards your chest to stretch your spine as much as possible without straining yourself .

*These exercise are very good   at stretching and
correcting any misalignments at the lumbar-
sacrum-iliac   joints.*

*%%%%%%%%%%%%%%%%%%%%%%%%%%%%%%
%%%%%%%%%*

*Rest   by taking   5 deep breaths in by
expanding your chest as much as possible and
exhaling slowly.*

*%%%%%%%%%%%%%%%%%%%%%%%%%%%%%%
%%%%%%%%%*

Exercise four

The moving bridge.

Lying down face up with your interlocked hand fingers under your head.
Bend your knees and raise your low back towards the ceiling and down to the mattress , up and down 10-20 times. Go easy and never strain yourself and as you get stronger increase the repetitions.

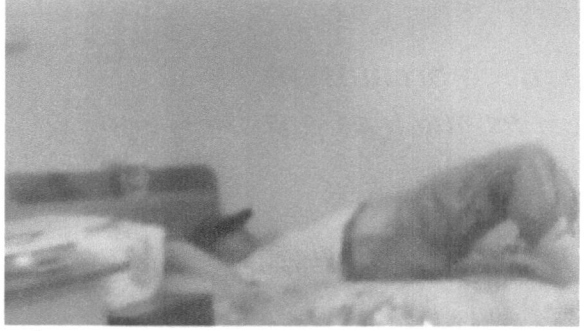

This exercise strengthens your abdominal , spinal and leg muscles and mobilizes the hip and sacroiliac joints.

$$ $$$$$$$$$$$

Rest   by taking 5 deep breaths in expanding your chest as much as possible and exhaling slowly.

@@@@@@@@@@@@@@@@@@@@@@@@@@@
@@@@@@@

Exercise five

Bend your right knee and bring it towards your chest and raise your head towards your knee. Repeat this exercise 5 times

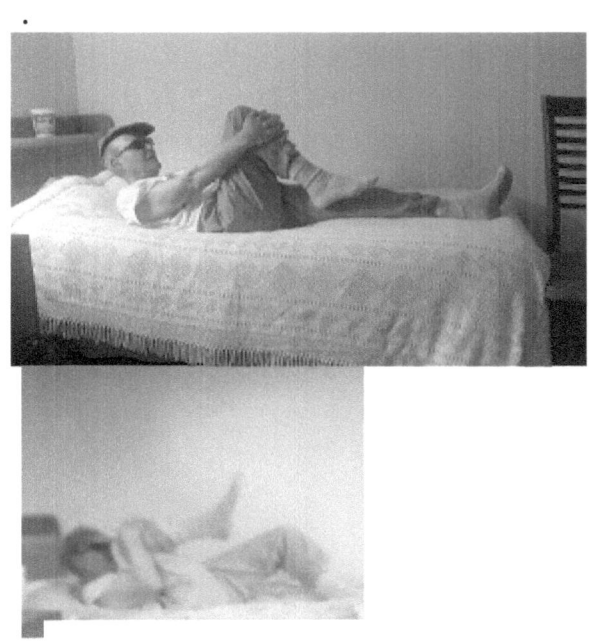

Repeat the same exercise with your left knee

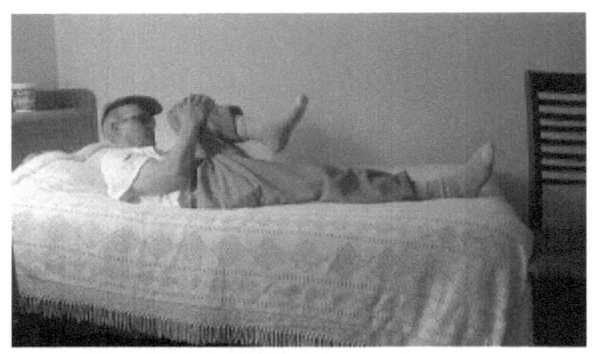

These exercises are very good to reduce any misalignments to the sacrum -iliac joints and sacrum lumbar vertebrae.. Also good for the abdominal muscles and good for all spinal joints stretch from the sacrum to the upper cervical vertebrae.

"This exercise makes positive changes in the joints, along with increasing the blood supply promoting healing by supplying necessary nutrients into the area."

@@@@@@@@@@@@@@@@@@@@@@@@@@@@@@@@@@@@
@@@@

Exercise six

Knees to chest exercises with   raising your head towards your knees.
Bend your knees and bring them to your chest as close as possible , without straining yourself
And raise your head towards your knees
Hold that position to the count of three
Repeat this exercise 5 times without straining yourself and as you get stronger you increase the repetitions by 1-2 every few days

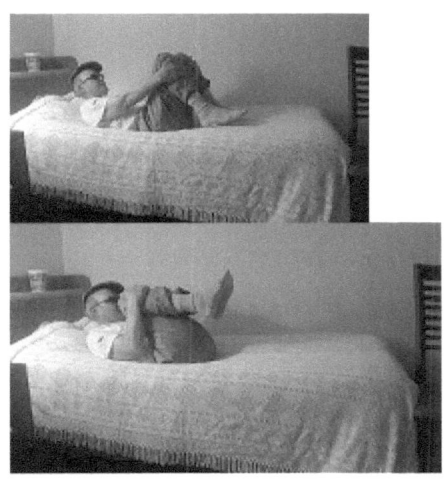

Go easy on yourself and do not over do it.

This exercise is good at mobilizing all the joints of your spine, hips and pelvis and increases the flexibility of the spine and   pelvis. It is a very good spinal stretch that increases the flexibility of the spine, increases the blood supply and promotes healing .

THIS IS A VERY IMPORTANT EXERCISE, AND THIS IS THE MAXIMUM (FLEXION) BEND FORWARD THAT MIMICS THE ADAMS TEST STRETCHING THE SPINE TO ITS MAXIMUM WITHOUT GRAVITY.

This exercise stretches the whole spine promoting good range of motion correcting any misalignments .

@@@@@@@@@@@@@@@@@@@@@@@@@@@@@
@@@@

Rest   by taking 5 deep breaths in expanding your chest as much as possible and exhaling slowly.

&&&&&&&&&&&&&&&&&&&&&&&&&&&&&

&&&&&&&

If there is any pain during the exercises, stop and rest, and do the exercises that are easy for you and pain free first.

Exercise seven

KNEES TO CHEST ROCKING EXERCISE

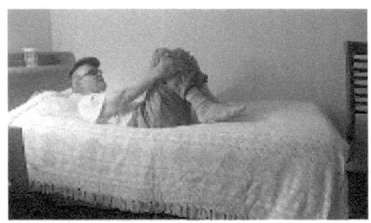

Knees to chest rocking
exercises :

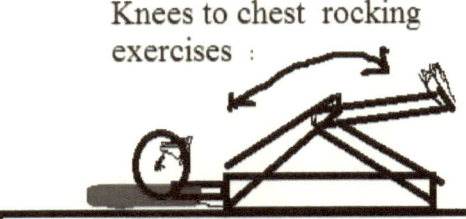

this is the most
important exercise
to increase the
flexibility of your
spine.

grab your right knee with your right
hand and your left knee with your left
hand and bring your knees to your
chest and with a rocking motion rock
your pelvis back and forth

*THIS EXERCISE MOBILIZES ALL JOINTS OF THE
SPINE, HIP
AND PELVIS JOINTS AND CHEST AND
SHOULDER JOINTS*

*Lying face up with your knees bent
And you hands at your side
Bring your bent knees towards your chest
Grab your right knee with your right hand*

And your left knee with your left hand

While holding your knees with your hands about 6- 12 inches apart

WITH A ROCKING MOVE

Rock your pelvis back and forth
by bringing your knees to your chest
And back without your feet touching the mat

Knees to chest rocking
exercises :

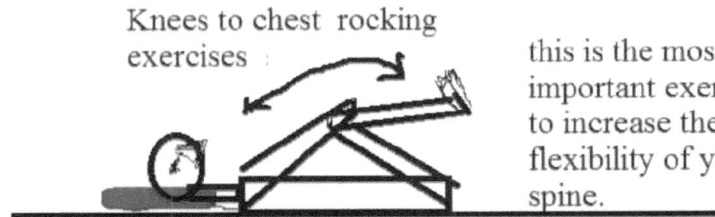

this is the most important exercise to increase the flexibility of your spine.

grab your right knee with your right hand and your left knee with your left hand and bring your knees to your chest and with a rocking motion rock your pelvis back and forth

REPEAT THIS EXERCISE 10-20 TIMES
WITHOUT STRAINING YOUR SELF

And increase the repetition every week by 5 until you reach 100 or more, depending on your physical condition and stamina.

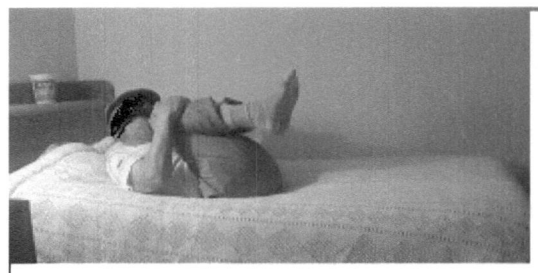

This exercise is very good at mobilizing all the joints of your spine, hips and pelvis, chest and shoulders.
Increases the flexibility of the spine and pelvis and strengthens the muscles of the spine. This exercise will correct any misalignments at the sacrum-lumbar - pelvis area and make those joints stronger.
Somebody suggested that this exercise promotes healing and regeneration on any damaged intervertebral disk disease.

Go easy on yourself and do not over do it, with time as you get stronger and more flexible you will be able to do more.
As your spine is getting stronger and more flexible the Cobb angle will be getting smaller and your spine straighter .

$$$$$$$$$$$$$$$$$$$$$$$$$$$$$$$$$$$
$$$$$$$$

Exercise 8

SACROILIAC SPINAL STRETCH

Lying face up , bend your right knee and let it down on the mat,
Your right foot is touching your left thigh.
Push your right knee downwards in the direction of your left foot,
Repeat 3-5 times on each knee

lying face up, bend
right knee and let it
down on right side on
mat

push your right knee
towards your other foot

Repeat this exercise 5 times

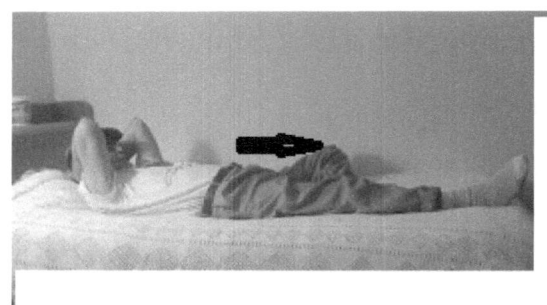

Repeat the same exercise on left side

*This exercise is stretching , mobilizing and
correcting the sacroiliac, and sacrum-L5 joints*

$$$
$$$$$$$$$$$$@@@@@@@@@@@@@@@@@@@@
@@@@@@@@@@@

Exercise nine

SPINAL STRETCH raising the head to chest with the hands behind the head

N.B. this is not a sit up exercise

Lying face up, hands behind the head,
Bring your elbows towards your face
And raise your head towards your chest without
straining yourself and then lower you head
gently to the mattress.
Repeat it 3-5 times and you can increase the
repetitions as you get stronger and more flexible

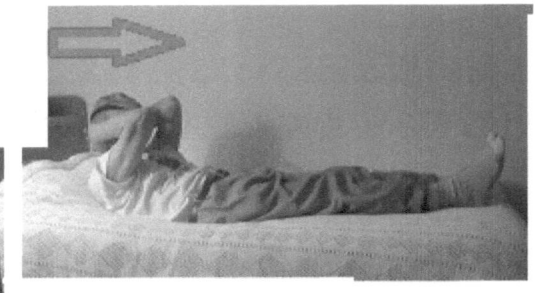

lying face up,hands behind the head
bring elbows towards the face
and raise your head towards your
chest and then gently down

*This exercise stretches and mobilizes the spinal
joints from the pelvis to the head.
Go easy and do not overdo it*

ⓐⓐⓐⓐⓐⓐⓐⓐⓐⓐⓐⓐⓐⓐⓐⓐⓐⓐⓐⓐⓐⓐⓐⓐ
ⓐⓐⓐⓐ

Exercise ten

*You finish with the same exercise as the number
one exercise*

Take a deep breath in
expanding your chest as
much as possible.
Exhale slowly. Repeat 5
times.

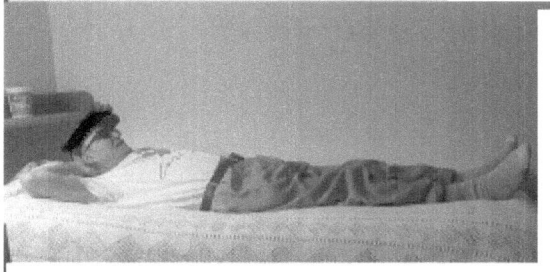

lying face up with your
handsbehindyour head
take a deep breath in expanding your
chest as much as possible
and then exhaling slowly
repeat X 5 times

This exercise is good for expanding your chest cavity stretching your ribs and your shoulder blades.. it will exercise, and strengthen the chest muscles . It will also mobilize and restore the normal range of motion to the ribs reducing any rib hump.

@@@@@@@@@@@@@@@@@@@@@@@@@@@
@@@@@

N.B. You do these exercises on an empty stomach and never after a meal, or a big drink.

YOU ALWAYS TAKE IT EASY AND NEVER STRAIN YOURSELF.

If some exercise causes pain , skip it and do another exercise until you are stronger and more flexible.

N.B. DO THESE EXERCISES 2- 3 TIMES A DAY UNLESS YOU ARE SICK OR HAVE FEVER IN WHICH CASE YOU DO NOT DO ANY EXERCISES

###
############

These are the exercises that have the potential to stop the progression of the abnormal spinal curves and even reverse the spine back to normal.

Of course there are more good exercises that have the potential to prevent and help you have a strong healthy and flexible spine.
Here are some of the best.
1)Swimming: swimming is an excellent exercise for preventing scoliosis and if you can swim , swim every time you have the chance. Fishes swim all the time and they never get scoliosis.

2)Monkey bar exercises are very good for stretching exercises of the spine. Spinal stretch or pull up exercises. The monkeys do these exercises all the time and they do not have any scoliosis.

3)Modified Adam's   forward bending test which I described in detailed in my book : how to prevent and treat scoliosis.

The modified Adam's forward bending test exercise is done by: START WITH THE STANDING POSITION
Your feet are placed 12 inches apart
Bend forwards from the waist without bending your knees
And touch your left foot   with your right fingers
While your left hand is at the back of your low back

Come up to straight position

And then bend forwards from your waist and touch your right foot with the fingers of your left hand
while your right hand is placed at your low back

N.B. if you have a noticeable rib hump on your right side,
Then do twice as many bends forwards with your right hand
To your left foot, and vice versa.

This is done because when you bend and bring your right hand(the same side of your rib hump) to your left foot,   the bending forwards stretches and brings forwards the rib hump and corrects your rib cage
And with time it should bring it back to its normal position.

That is why you do the forwards bends twice as much on the side of the rib hump.

START WITH THE STANDING POSITION BUT
YOUR FEET ARE PLACED 12-18 INCHES APART
BEND FORWARDS AND TOUCH YOUR LEFT
FOOT WTIH YOUR RIGHT HAND FINGERS
WHILE YOUR LEFT HAND RESTS ON THE BACK
OF YOUR LOW BACK

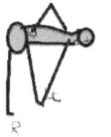

Here is the summary of the spinal active flexion exercises with pictures

LIE FACE UP
ON A MAT OR
A MATRESS

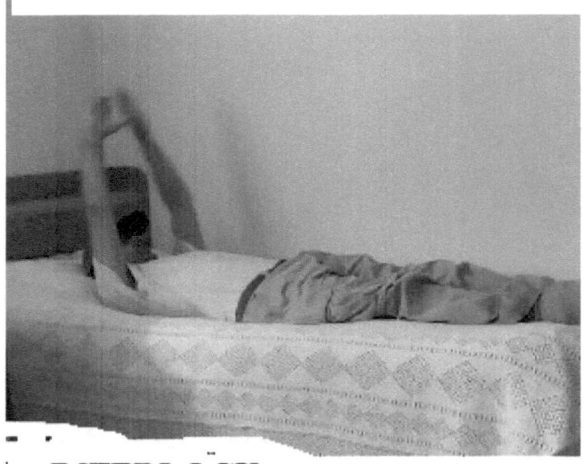

INTERLOCK
YOUR FINGERS
AND PLACE
THEM UNDER
YOUR HEAD

Positioning for the exercises

lie face up interlock your
hands and place them
under your head

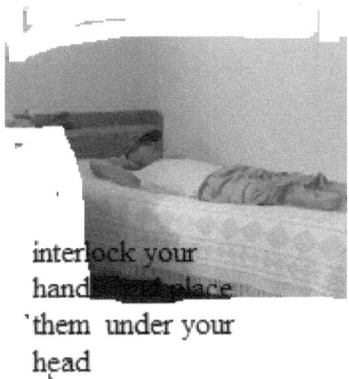

interlock your
hands and place
them under your
head

Take a deep breath in
expanding your chest as
much as possible.
Exhale slowly. Repeat 5
times.

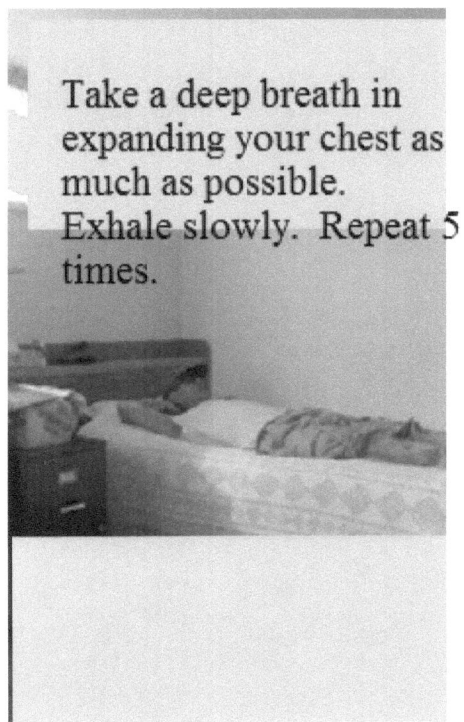

lying face up,
interlock fingers
and place them
under your head

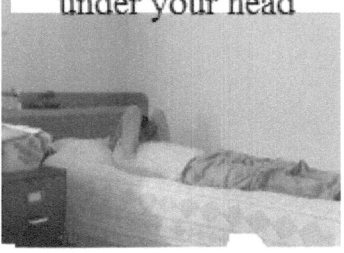

bring your elbows
towards your face ,
then back pressing on
the mattress

Breathing exercises
face and back

bent elbows to

pressing on the

mattress

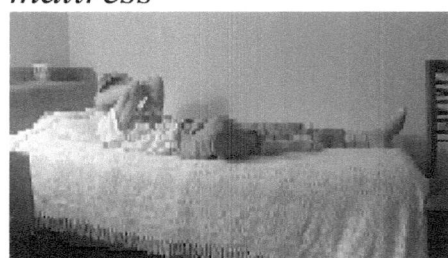

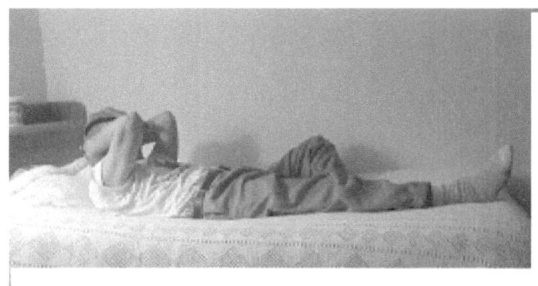

Knee to the side and raise the head to chest

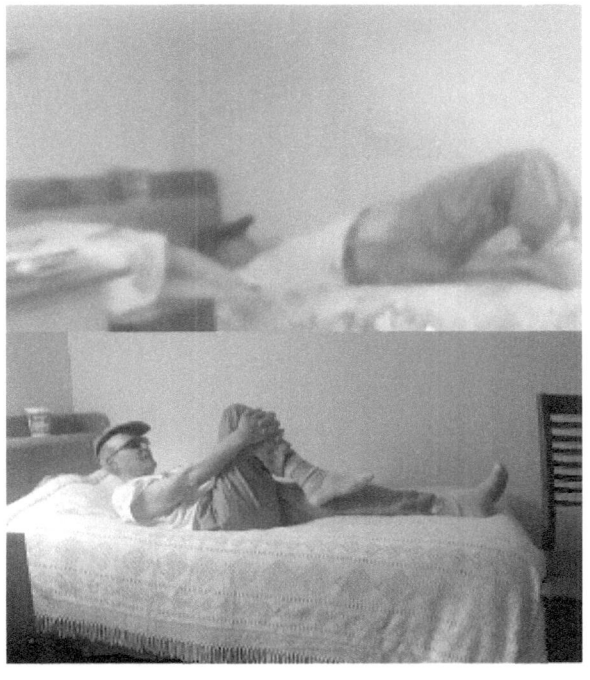

The moving bridge exercise   *bend your knee and bring to*
Raise your low back up and down   *your chest*

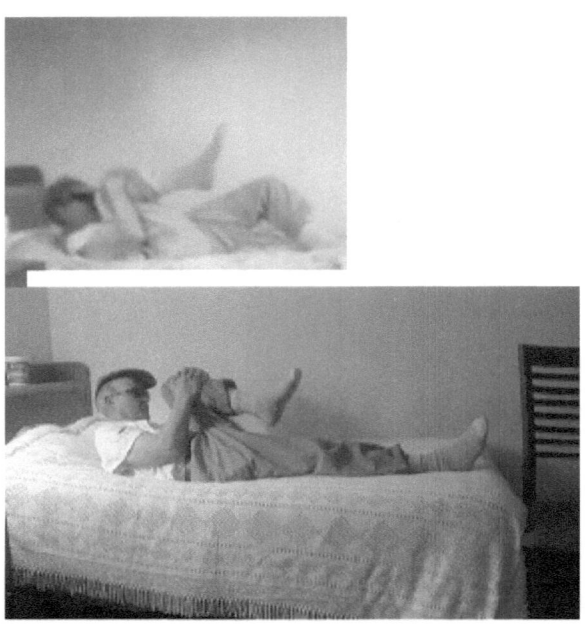

Knee to chest exercises

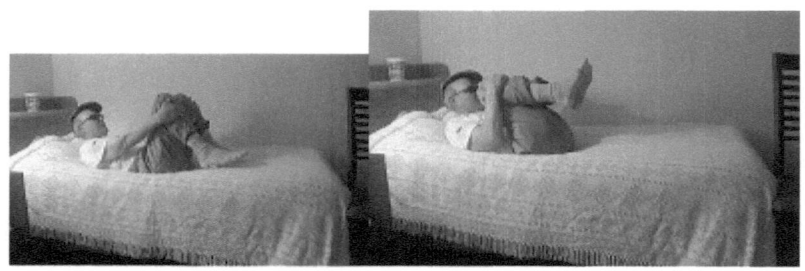

Knees to chest and raising head towards the knees

Knees to chest rocking
exercises :

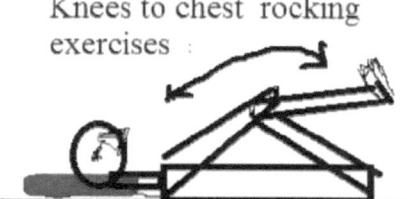

this is the most
important exercise
to increase the
flexibility of your
spine.

grab your right knee with your right
hand and your left knee with your left
hand and bring your knees to your
chest and with a rocking motion rock
your pelvis back and forth

lying face up, bend
right knee and let it
down on right side on
mat

push your right knee
towards your other foot

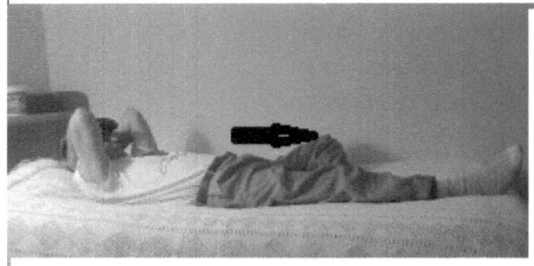

*Knee to the side and push the knee down towards
the other foot*

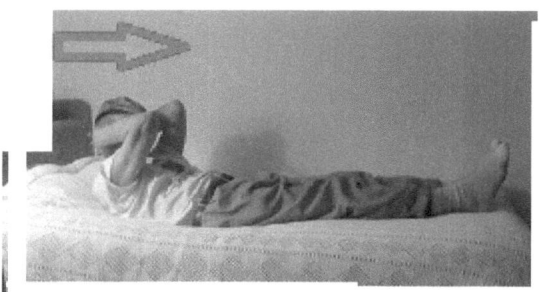

lying face up, hands behind the head
bring elbows towards the face
and raise your head towards your
chest and then gently down

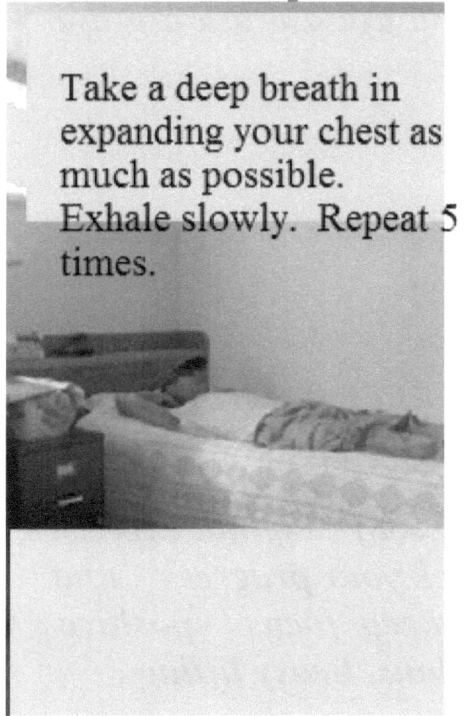

Take a deep breath in
expanding your chest as
much as possible.
Exhale slowly. Repeat 5
times.

Bring   Both bent elbows   to   deep breathing
exercises
the face and raise the head

To the chest X5

ⓐⓐⓐⓐⓐⓐⓐⓐⓐⓐⓐⓐⓐⓐⓐⓐⓐⓐⓐⓐⓐⓐⓐⓐⓐⓐⓐ
ⓐⓐⓐⓐⓐ

20) *FOR BETTER RESULTS KEEP A DAILY DIARY.*

When you start doing the s.a.f.e. spinal exercises keep a daily diary to check your progress and the most important is to keep focus , positive and avoid slouching positions, heavy lifting , especially heavy babies.

Take a picture of your spine just before starting

the exercises and re-take pictures of your spine every week to see the progress you are making.

You should see some improvements in your spine in 4-6 weeks and as the time goes by, your spine will be stronger and more flexible. Any abnormal curves will start to improve and reduced.

Everyday write down exactly how you do the exercises, how many times you do each exercise and how you feel during and after the exercises.

Remember never to strain yourself or overdo it, and as you get stronger and more flexible increase the repetitions of each exercise.

THE DAILY DIARY WILL MOTIVATE AND ENCOURAGE YOU WHEN YOU START SEEING IMPROVEMENTS IN YOUR SCOLIOSIS.

As time goes by and you feel stronger increase the repetitions
And the time you do them. More repetitions means stronger muscles and more flexible spine.

The most important is that you do these exercises to get better , healthier, more flexibility and above

*all to stop the progression of any abnormal
curves and reduce   the angle of your scoliosis.*

*Even when your spine feels better and your
scoliosis is reduced, keep doing these exercises at
least once a day to keep your spine strong, healthy
and flexible.*

*Get into the habit to do them every morning
when you get up before you have any breakfast.*

*Always remember that exercises and good
nutrition is the mother of good health, good
posture and longevity with good quality of life.*

@@@@@@@@@@@@@@@@@@@@@@@@@
@@@

21)EXPECTED RESULTS

The S.A.F.E .   exercises are designed to give

flexibility and strength to the spine as long as you do them daily.

To have good results you have to change your old habits of bad posture at home, at school and avoid slouching everywhere else.

If you do the exercises and keep doing what you have been doing that started the scoliosis, do not expect much, because you did not remove the CAUSE, 'the bad postural habits" that started the scoliosis in the first place.

You might see some improvement but not as much as when you removed the cause, the bad posture habits and lifting of heavy objects including heavy babies or school bags.

if you do the exercises daily three times a day and you removed the cause of the scoliosis, and if you are a girl you should stop lifting and carrying babies around *, With these exercises along with some swimming exercises and monkey bar stretching exercises you should get good results in 2-3 months . These exercises should stop the progression of the abnormal curve called scoliosis and the Cobb angle of your scoliosis should start* to get smaller and smaller with time.

That will depend on the effort you put into the
exercises and your avoidance of what causes the
scoliosis, such as lifting heavy objects, slouching,
when you sit at home, in class and walking.

Even when you see some improvement you
should keep doing the exercises daily for ever . if
you want to have a strong ,healthy, flexible spine,
along with all the other health benefits that come
with a healthy spine, like good health, good looks
and good posture.
The exercises will be taking you about 15 minutes
times 3 a total of 45 minutes a day and the health
benefits are enormous . Besides you do not
waste time going to a gym and you need no
equipment to do the exercises.

Of course you will be doing these exercises on an
empty stomach and you should not exercise when
you are sick with fever , infections or have severe
pain.

I am not a fun or believer of "NO PAIN NO
GAIN." slogan.
When there is pain, it is a warning from your
body to stop and you should always listen to your
body. DO the exercises that do not cause any pain

and gradually do more. Let your body guide you what exercises are suitable for you!

@@@@@@@@@@@@@@@@@@@@@@@@@@@@@@@@
@@@@

@@@@@@@@@@@@@@@@@@@@@@@@@@@@@@@@
@@@@

22)EXERCISES TO PREVENT SCOLIOSIS

If you are lucky enough and you do not have scoliosis, count your blessings but it is a good idea to do some spinal exercises and other exercises to prevent any abnormal curves of your spine.

Besides , exercises and good nutrition is the mother of good health and everyone should exercise daily to have good health and a strong healthy flexible spine without any abnormal curves by any name.

Here are a few spinal exercises that are good for everyone to do daily to prevent scoliosis and other spinal curves.

1)Both knees to chest exercises done every day especially in the morning before you eat.

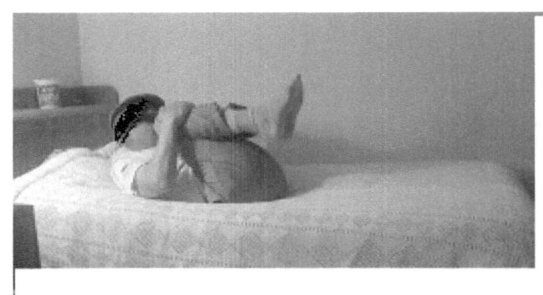

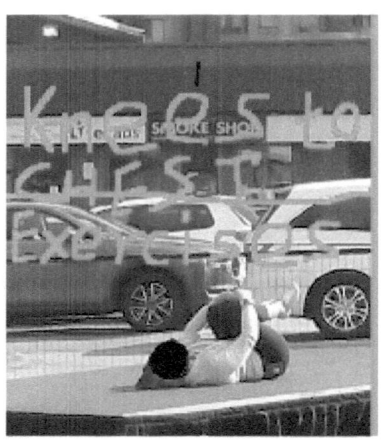

2)knees to chest rocking exercises.

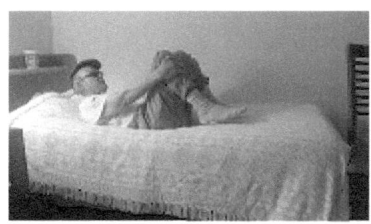

Knees to chest rocking
exercises : 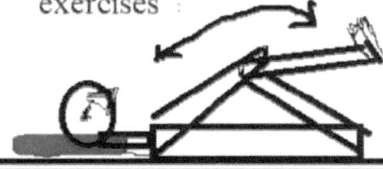 this is the most
important exercise
to increase the
flexibility of your
spine.

grab your right knee with your right
hand and your left knee with your left
hand and bring your knees to your
chest and with a rocking motion rock
your pelvis back and forth

*3)raising your head to your chest with the hands
interlocked behind your head . This is not a sit up
exercise .*

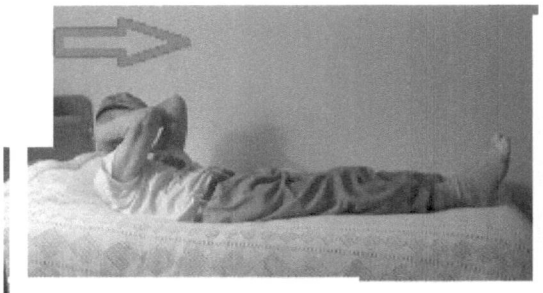

lying face up, hands behind the head
bring elbows towards the face
and raise your head towards your
chest and then gently down

4)single knee to chest exercise X5 times on each knee

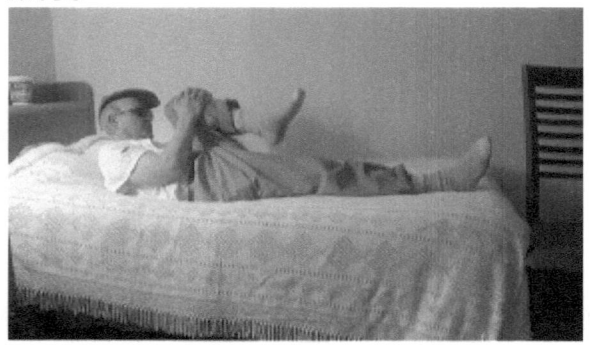

Other good exercises are swimming, walking without slouching,
And monkey bar exercises.

These are all spinal stretching exercises that make

the spine strong, healthy and flexible safeguarding the spine from any injuries or abnormal curves.

Besides prevention is better than any treatment.

@@@@@@@@@@@@@@@@@@@@@@@@
@@@@@

23) WHAT EXERCISES YOU SHOULD AVOID

Good exercises will make your spine strong, healthy, flexible and will safeguard your spine from any injury.

Bad exercises will have the potential to cause injury to the spine and even cause chronic debilitating diseases.

Avoid any exercise that requires twisting and bending.
Avoid all extension and twisting exercises. They can cause injuries to the spine and the beginning of scoliosis at any age,

Avoid lifting exercises unless you have a low back support and you bend your knees.
Stop any exercise that cause pain. Pain is a warning that whatever you do is not good for the body.
Avoid any warm up stretches that require bending and twisting or any spinal extension stretching.
Avoid any dancing dips and the limbo dance which is bad for the spine.
Avoid any exercise that requires you to be in a bad uncomfortable postural position.
Always go easy on any new exercises. Give your body a chance to get used to them.
Avoid any exercises that require to go beyond the normal range of a joint. Do not press your luck. You risk to injure that joint.

Avoid any head stands. You can easily injure your neck and the rest of your body if you fall the wrong way. Your neck is not made to support your

whole body, but just your head.
Avoid any spinal extension exercises especially if you scoliosis, it makes the curve worse.

&&&&&&&&&&&&&&&&&&&&&&&&&&&&&&&&&&&&&&&&&&&&&&&&&&&

24)Scoliosis & Nutrition

Nutrition Is always a factor for good health. As I mention above , according to an English study, the congenital scoliosis is caused by a deficiency of folic acid, and now the doctors advice their pregnant patients to supplement their diets with folic acid to prevent any abnormality or other malformations and bony defects to the unborn baby.
There are some writings that they try to link idiopathic scoliosis to some minerals deficiencies such as selenium, copper and other minerals but there is no conclusive evidence to that. If the were talking about calcium deficiency and vitamin D, that would be reasonable and we are going to talk about it later in this chapter. As calcium and vitamin D is the cornerstone of healthy bones. As usual there are many theories about everything but

they are just theories. Besides , scoliosis is a structural problem caused by some injury to the sacral-lumbar-iliac area. I consider such theories, just theories without any concrete proof. If that was the case the doctors would just prescribe selenium or whatever and that would be the end of scoliosis. But that is not happening and nobody takes such theories seriously.

However we know that poor nutrition can lead to many diseases, deformities and conditions.. Rickets, the most common childhood disease in developing countries, it is a softening of the bones due to deficiency or impaired metabolism of vitamin D, phosphorus and calcium, potentially leading to fractures and deformity. In rare cases it can occur in adults too but the majority of cases occur in children suffering from severe malnutrition, usually resulting from famine or starvation during the early stages of childhood.. When it occurs in adults is called Osteomalacia and it is also due to a deficiency of vitamin D and calcium.
An extreme and prolonged vitamin D deficiency can cause Rickets which is the softening and weakening of bones in children.
Vitamin D promotes the absorption of calcium and phosphorus from the gastrointestinal tract and a deficiency of vitamin D makes it difficult to maintain proper calcium and phosphorus levels in

bones, which causes rickets.

Signs and symptoms of rickets can include:
 Delayed growth ,Pain in the spine, pelvis and legs ,Muscle weakness, Bowed legs or knock knees Thickened wrists and ankles

Breastbone projection .Because rickets softens the growth plates at the ends of a child's bones, it can cause skeletal deformities.

The complications of rickets are , failure to grow, abnormally curved spine, (scoliosis), dental defects, seizures and other skeletal deformities.

The cause of rickets as we mention above is vitamin D deficiency and Occasionally, not getting enough calcium or lack of calcium and vitamin D can cause rickets.

As we can see vitamin D calcium deficiency has the potential to cause abnormalities to the skeletal system including scoliosis, but there will be the obvious signs and symptoms of the rickets disease. For the prevention of rickets ,provide the kids with vitamin D and calcium . Vitamin D can be produced by the human skin when it is exposed to sunlight and from foods like eggs, fish oil , milk and other foods that are fortified with vitamin D.

It is sad in this day and age ,that even in rich countries there are malnourished kids suffering form rickets and other diseases from the lack of proper nutrition.
 In my book :

EAT THE RIGHT FOODS FOR OPTIMUM HEALTH

Publish by amazon.com and available in both eBook and print form.

In that book I emphasized that good nutrition is essential for everybody to have optimum health. And the father of medicine wrote: "Let food be thy medicine and medicine be thy food" ~Hippocrates. So it is necessary to provide all the nutrients for the body to function properly.

I recommend that all my readers have a good nutritional diet and exercise daily to keep their bodies in good health. For all the kids in the growing years it is good to have milk fortified with vitamin D , eggs fruits and vegetables daily for good health and to prevent any nutritional deficiencies.

Good nutrition and daily exercises is the mother of good health!

And here are some quotes about health and nutrition.

"QUOTES ABOUT HEALTH AND NUTRITION

The greatest wealth is Health." ~Unknown

Eating smart will not only make you smart, it's the smart thing to do.
Eating right does wonders for your body.

"If you don't take care of your body, where are you going to live?" ~Unknown
"Take care of your body. It's the only place you have to live."

25) If you have scoliosis

If you are diagnosed with scoliosis, you should know that you are not alone suffering from this condition. Unfortunately, there are millions of people suffering from this condition. Some of them worse than others. The bigger the Cobb angle is the worse the scoliosis is.

The most important thing to remember is " that is not your fault." This can happen to anyone at any time for different reasons.

The most important thing you can do is start exercising to stop the progression of the abnormal curve while it is still small, manageable and can be reversed. The sooner you start the better your

chances to reduce the scoliosis while it is still small and manageable.

Unfortunately there is no magic pill to take and make the scoliosis disappear .With the spinal exercises you will have a good chance to stop the progression of the abnormal curve and even reverse it back to a healthy spine.

Do not expect miracles to happen overnight , but if you have the will, desire and determination to do the exercises daily in the privacy of your home even in your own bed or just a mat on the floor of your house, you will have a good chance to get a strong and healthy spine without any abnormal curve called scoliosis.

If you want to get better and stop the abnormal curve from becoming bigger you have to do the exercises. NOBODY ELSE CAN DO THESE EXERCISES FOR YOU.

IT IS YOUR CHOICE, you do the exercises and you get better or you do nothing and your scoliosis might get worse.

So far "the wait and see approach" used by many health professionals did not work well for the people suffering from scoliosis and many end up with surgery and rods in their spine.

If you have pain in your low back along with scoliosis , use an elastic spinal support under your clothes to protect your spine for any further injury. Or you can use one of those corset

garment that the women use to wear for spinal protection and
Good posture. Of course you remove the support

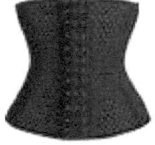

CORSET

during the exercises.

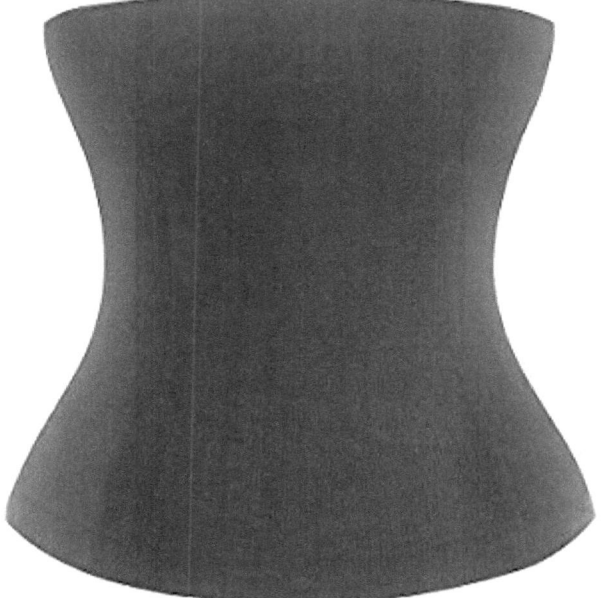

You probably do not need a bulky and expensive spinal brace. A fashionable cheap corset might as well do the same job as an expensive spinal brace. The idea is to support your spine until your spine is strong and flexible with the S.A.F.E. exercises you will be doing.
If you decide to use a corset buy one that will give you a good support of your sacroiliac joints .

There are no guarantees in life, but you will have a good chance to help your self if you have the will, desire and determination to reduce your curve by doing the spinal active flexion exercises daily.

N.B. If the scoliosis is due to pathology or severe trauma ,
or you had surgery with rods in your spine, these exercises are not for you. If that's your case consult your attending doctor for proper treatments and exercise recommendations.

@@@@@@@@@@@@@@@@@@@@@@@@@@@@

26)For the professionals diagnosing and treating scoliosis.

I am sure all the health professionals are doing their best to help their patients and I commend them for that . Many times them are frustrated or disappointed for not getting as good results with their treatments and procedures as they wish to get.

As they know, SCOLIOSIS is called IDIOPATHIC, meaning that there is no known cause for the abnormal spinal curve and by not knowing the cause, the treatments are not effective.

However scoliosis has not only one cause but many causes .

As they know the base of the human frame is the feet, so if one foot is shorter than the other it will cause an imbalance to the human frame and will cause an abnormal tilt of the pelvis causing a curve the so called scoliosis . So it is always a good idea to check the length of the feet first, and if there is a true short leg, they have to fix that first with a heel lift or a shoe lift . No matter what they do to that patient, will not be effective without the correction of the feet length .That is absolutely necessary to correct the cause of that scoliosis which is the true short leg.

If the feet are equal, then they have to look at the second base of the human frame which is the pelvis and the sacrum. Any tilt to the pelvis and sacrum which is the base of the spine will cause a primary abnormal curve starting at the lumbar-sacral area and a secondary curve in the thoracic spine due to the righting reflex, where the body tries to bring the centre of gravity within the base of the human frame. The x-rays will confirm the origin of the abnormal curve , the scoliosis.

The cause of that abnormal pelvis tilt at the lumbar -sacral .Ilium joints usually is from a lifting accident, lifting something heavy, a fall, or bending and twisting. In the case of the girls scoliosis, the cause is the lifting of heavy babies. It can also be from bad postural habits, bad positioning of the body over a period of time.

In order to have good results with any treatment you have to eliminate the cause, the lifting of heavy objects and replace the bad postural habits with good postural habits. .

As soon as a diagnosis is made they have to initiate and remove the causes and initiate corrective measures to rehabilitate the lumbar-sacral pelvis area. A small elastic support in the low back for protection is also advisable for a short period of time.

The wait and see approach is a waste of valuable time and in the meantime a small manageable scoliosis become severe and more difficult to treat.

I suggest, (and it is just a suggestion I cannot tell anybody how to do their job) to replace the wait and see approach or as is now called "OBSERVATION PERIOD" with "THE ACTION TO STOP THE ABNORMAL CURVE OF SCOLIOSIS FROM GETTING WORSE" . By removing the cause or in other words the bad habits of the youngsters and the lifting of heavy objects, the abnormal curve will stop from getting worse.

Then they have to instruct their patients to start exercising with the right exercises to correct any misalignment in the low back joints and make the spine stronger, healthier, more flexible .

The S.A.F.E. exercises or other suitable exercises, are the "ONE STITCH IN TIME TO SAVE NINE" , they have the potential to stop a mild scoliosis from becoming a severe scoliosis requiring, braces and surgery with spinal fusion and rods in the spine . The exercises will make the spine strong and more flexible without any abnormal curves.

Find the cause, fix the cause or eliminate the cause and exercise to have strong spinal muscles and a flexible spine.

The millions of people that exercise daily prove that exercising and good nutrition is the mother of good health. They have strong healthy and flexible spines and no scoliosis.

27)Conclusion

Every year millions of people are diagnosed with scoliosis and most of them are girls in their growing years. The reason why girls are affected more than the boys with scoliosis is their motherhood instinct.   From an early age they want to prepare for the biggest role of their lives when they become mothers themselves. They want to sharpen their skills how to take care of kids, their siblings, cousins nephews and even the kids of neighbors. They play and lift the kids carrying them around pretending that they are their mothers and take care of them. By lifting the kids and carrying them around they injure their low backs, sacral-lumbar area setting them up for the development of an abnormal curve in the lumbar area and if left undiagnosed and untreated a secondary curve develops in the thoracic spine above due to the righting reflex.

Unfortunately nothing can change the motherhood instinct of girls and girls will continue to play and lift other heavy kids and the will be getting scoliosis. What we can do , we can educate the parents and their doctors to recognize the cause of scoliosis that it is a lifting or strain injury to the low back. By recognizing the cause early and treat it properly with corrective actions it will stop a mild scoliosis from becoming a severe curve requiring surgery and rods in their spines.

Everybody has the potential to get an injury by lifting heavy objects, falling down or anything that can injure the low back and if left untreated it will become chronic and will cause some abnormal curve in the spine which is called scoliosis. For the girls and the boys the injury is more serious and most of the time is unreported and untreated or poorly treated and that is the cause of their severe scoliosis.

In this book I tried to raise the awareness of the cause of scoliosis in girls , boys and everybody else. It is the injury, strain , sprain or whatever you want to call it, to the low back pelvis-sacral and sacral-lumbar joints. The MOTHER of scoliosis , as I see the injuries to these lumbar-sacral-iliac area, By recognizing the cause and eliminating the cause and exercising with the spinal active flexion exercises S.A.F.E.   it will stop the progression of scoliosis and even reverse it back to normal. By doing so, it will reduce the number of people having debilitating severe scoliosis affecting their health, and they will have a better quality of life .

It should be early diagnosis, early treatment and no wasting precious time with the so called observation period.

&&&&&&&&&&&&&&&&&&&&&&&&&&&
&&&&&&&&&&&&&&&&&&&&&&&&&&&&
&&&&&&&&&&&&&&&&&&&&&&&

28) Epilog

Scoliosis is a preventable and treatable structural condition of the spine. Millions of youngsters are diagnosed with mild idiopathic scoliosis every year in all parts of the world and some of these youngsters are going to develop severe scoliosis

*requiring surgery and other treatments during
their lifetime. It is an epidemic affecting the quality
of life of those affected by scoliosis. The purpose of
this book is to educate people that with the
necessary precautions, scoliosis can be avoided.
Avoiding bad postural habits and lifting injuries
will keep scoliosis at bay. Even if after all the
precautions an injury occur to the low back or
from bad postural habits and a mild scoliosis
develops with an early diagnosis and the proper
treatments a severe scoliosis can be avoided.
It is absolutely necessary when the initial
diagnosis of scoliosis is made and the abnormal
curve is small , to replace the usual "PERIOD OF
OBSERVATION" and the loss of precious time
with the "PERIOD OF ACTION " to stop the
progression of the abnormal curve . An early
diagnosis and treatment of scoliosis with the
necessary support of the affected area and the one
stitch in time, the spinal active flexion exercises
,S.A.F.E, to stop the progression of the abnormal
curve and even reverse it back to normal.
It will be even better, if all people young and old,
girls and boys take preventative measures to avoid
any spinal abnormal curves by exercising daily
with the spinal active flexion exercises(S.A.F.E)
to have a strong, healthy and flexible spine. All
the athletes of the world, are doing similar or a
variation of these exercises daily and they have*

no scoliosis.
When everybody exercises and take the necessary
precautions, Girls , boys and everybody else can
avoid a lifelong suffering from the devastating
effects of the abnormal curve called scoliosis!

@@@@@@@@@@@@@@@@@@@@@@@
@@@@@@@

29)References

1) *congenital scoliosis cause:" Jan 26, 2007Allen J. Wilcox, M.D., Ph.D., lead NIEHS author on the new study published online in the British Medical Journal. "*

2) **A Dangerous Curve: The Role of History in America's Scoliosis Screening Programs**

3) **ADAMS TEST**

4) **Children Born with Addiction Why Does It Happen & How Is ...**
*https://www.addictionhelper.com/**children/born-***

with-addiction-why-and-how-it-is-treated

5) " _**Thalidomide - A Drug That Malformed Thousands of People**_
https://www.englishonline.at/health_medicine/**thali domide/thalidomide**-victims.htm

6) *SCOLIOSIS*:
A FRESH LOOK AT WHAT CAUSES THE IDIOPATHIC FUNCTIONAL SCOLIOSIS AND HOME EXERCISES TO STOP THE PROGRESSION OF THE CURVE AND EVEN REVERSE IT BACK TO NORMAL
By S.ELIA

For the back cover of the book

Scoliosis is a preventable condition and unfortunately it can affect anyone at any age. Usually the youngsters and especially the girls are affected more than others.

In this book you will learn why the girls are affected with scoliosis more often than the boys. In this book you will learn what is causing the abnormal curve called scoliosis and how to remove that cause so that the treatments are effective in reversing the scoliosis.

In this book you will learn what exercises are good to stop the progression of scoliosis and even to reverse it.

In this book you will learn how to prevent scoliosis with the right exercises so that your spine is strong, healthy and flexible.

Read the book and take action to prevent and treat the idiopathic scoliosis with the s.a.f.e. spinal exercises.

Even if you do not have scoliosis   by reading this book you will learn what exercises are good to prevent scoliosis.

Read the book and find out what exercises you should avoid.

Read this book to find out what causing the congenital scoliosis and how to prevent it by taking the right supplements.

Read this book to find out how to protect your low back from injury, in your every day life.

In short this book is for every one that has a spine, and the spine is the backbone for good health.

Read this book to take good care of your spine and

your precious health!
When buying this book, consider it as a small
investment for you health especially your spine.
This small investment might save you money and
time in the long run by keeping you HEALTHY!

A healthy spine is THE KEY for a healthy body and
mind.

N.B. The exercises in this book are not intended
for people with severe trauma, pathology or had
surgery and rods in their spine.
if that's the case consult with your doctor for
proper treatments.

S.ELIA